The No B.S. Guide to Postpartum Care

Quick Recovery and Emotional Wellness Without the Stress

Eliza Kindler

Table of Contents

INTRODUCTION: WELCOME TO MOTHERHOOD 1

CHAPTER 1: UNDERSTANDING THE FOURTH TRIMESTER.................................. 5

THE FOURTH TRIMESTER. 5
    Fourth Trimester for Babies 6
PHYSICAL CHANGES 7
EMOTIONS AND MENTAL HEALTH 9
    Emotional Aspects for Moms.. 10
    Emotional Aspects for Babies 11
COMMON CHALLENGES 12

CHAPTER 2: PHYSICAL RECOVERY AFTER CHILDBIRTH 15

AFTER DELIVERY.. 15
    What to Expect 16
    Self-Care 18
    Pain Management.. 19
    Alternative Therapies... 20
    Natural Remedies 23
    Exercises and Stretches.. 24
    Postpartum Recovery Tips 26
    Rest and Self-Care... 27
WARNING SIGNS 29

CHAPTER 3: EMOTIONAL WELL-BEING AND MENTAL HEALTH 31

UNDERSTANDING THE BABY BLUES 32
    Why Do New Mothers Feel So Down? 33
    Could Your Partner Have the Baby Blues?.......................... 33
    Coping Strategies.. 34
IDENTIFYING AND MANAGING PPD 34
    Recognizing Signs and Symptoms.................................. 35
    Strategies for Managing PPD 37
    PPD Self-Assessment Quiz... 37
SEEKING SUPPORT 42
    PPD 42
    PNA 43
    Where to Find Support.. 44
    Benefits of Individual Counseling................................ 45

Benefits of Group Therapy 45

Online Resources 45

SELF-CARE PRACTICES FOR EMOTIONAL WELL-BEING 46

Relaxation Techniques 46

Mindfulness Exercises 47

Journaling 47

Prioritizing Personal Needs 47

Warning Against Burnout 47

CHAPTER 4: OPTIMAL NUTRITION FOR RECOVERY AND WELL-BEING 49

POSTPARTUM DIETARY REQUIREMENTS...50

Additional Calories 50

Protein 51

Essential Nutrients for Recovery and Lactation......................................52

Superfoods for Healing and Energy 54

Things to Avoid When Breastfeeding 56

MEAL PLANNING AND PREPARATION TIPS...57

Sample Meal Plan...58

SUPPLEMENTS 59

Calcium Supplements 60

Vitamin D Supplements 60

Iron Supplements..60

CHAPTER 5: BREASTFEEDING 101—FROM CHALLENGES TO SUCCESS 63

COMMON BREASTFEEDING CHALLENGES AND SOLUTIONS 64

Low Milk Supply..64

Engorgement (Stiff, Sore, and Painful Breast Swelling)..............................65

Mastitis and Fungal Infections 66

Sore Nipples...67

Inverted, Flat, or Huge Nipples 68

Tongue-Tie..68

Baby Gassy or Fussy After Feeding 68

LATCHING AND POSITIONING TECHNIQUES 69

Positioning..69

Step-by-Step Guide to Achieving a Good Latch 72

BREAST CARE AND PUMPING ADVICE 73

Storing Breast Milk...75

FEEDING ALTERNATIVES...76

Combi Feeding: Combining Breastfeeding and Formula Feeding................77

Deconstructing the "Breast Is Best" Myth 78

CHAPTER 6: NEWBORN CARE ESSENTIALS 81

NEWBORN HYGIENE AND DIAPERING 81

Bathing Your Newborn 82

Umbilical Cord Care 82
Proper Diaper Care 83
Cutting Your Baby's Nails.. 83
Oral Hygiene 84
Handling Visitors.. 84
SLEEPING AND SOOTHING TECHNIQUES 84
Establishing Healthy Sleep Patterns 86
Creating a Soothing Sleep Environment 86
Soothing Techniques for a Fussy Baby.. 86
RECOGNIZING AND ADDRESSING COMMON ISSUES 88
Colic 89
Gas.. 89
Reflux.. 90
Jaundice 90
Cow's Milk Protein Allergy 91
Respiratory Distress 91

CHAPTER 7: PARENTING WITH CONFIDENCE 93

BONDING WITH YOUR CHILD.. 94
How Infants Form Bonds 94
Various Parent–Child Bonding Activities.. 95
ESTABLISHING ROUTINES AND SCHEDULES.. 97
Benefits of Routines... 98
Practical Tips for Establishing Routines 99
BEING PRESENT 100
Being Physically Present With Your Baby 101
Being Mentally Present With Your Baby... 102
Being Spiritually Present With Your Baby 103
AVOIDING COMPARISONS 103
The Risks of Comparing Your Child to Others 104

CHAPTER 8: RETURNING TO WORK 107

PLANNING FOR CHILDCARE... 108
Researching and Visiting Potential Childcare Options.................... 108
Considering Cost and Availability 108
MANAGING TIME AND PRIORITIES 112
Setting Boundaries.. 113
Learning to Delegate Tasks 113
Recognizing the Need for Flexibility... 113
Simplifying Your Meal Plans 113
Scheduling Your Household Chores 114
Establishing Fixed Working Hours 114
Setting Achievable Daily Goals 114
Remembering to Have Some Fun! 114

Recognizing the Significance of Self-Care *115*
Maintaining Personal Fulfillment and Identity *115*
BUILDING A SUPPORT NETWORK *116*
Importance of Seeking Support *116*
Guidance on Building a Support Network *117*
Building and Nurturing Your Inner Circle *117*
Creating and Nurturing Your Outer Circle *118*

CHAPTER 9: SELF-CARE AND WELLNESS FOR MOTHERS **119**

MANAGING STRESS *120*
Be Aware of Your Expectations...*120*
Consider Exercise for Stress Release *121*
Don't Expect Too Much of Yourself...*121*
Stop Comparing Yourself to Others *121*
Reach Out and Connect With Friends, Family, and Professionals *121*
Be Aware of How Much Stress You Are Under and How Long You Have Felt This Way *122*
EXERCISE AND PHYSICAL ACTIVITY *122*
Benefits of Exercise..*123*
Safe and Effective Postpartum Exercises *123*
EMBRACING BODY POSITIVITY *124*
Strategies to Promote Self-Esteem and a Positive Body Image.................*125*
Self-Compassion Is Essential...*127*
Nutrition and Exercise as Forms of Self-Regulation....................................*127*

CHAPTER 10: BEYOND THE FOURTH TRIMESTER **129**

LONG-TERM PHYSICAL AND EMOTIONAL WELL-BEING *130*
Tips for Long-Term Health After the Postpartum Period...........................*131*
Addressing Lingering Concerns..*132*
Balancing Act..*132*
PLANNING FOR FUTURE PREGNANCIES *132*
Risks of Close Pregnancy Spacing *133*
Risks of Spacing Pregnancies Too Far Apart..*134*
Best Interval Between Pregnancies *134*
Birth Control Options...*135*
Return of Periods *136*
LEARNING, RESOURCES, AND SUPPORT...*137*
Importance of Continuous Growth *138*

CONCLUSION **139**

KEY TAKEAWAYS *140*
A CALL TO ACTION *142*

APPENDIX: BABY FOOD—SIX TO TWELVE MONTHS.................................... **143**

Signs Your Baby Is Ready for Solids 143
Critical Guidelines for Introducing Solid Foods 144
Suitable Foods........... 145
    Foods at Six Months.. 145
    Foods at Seven to Eight Months 146
    Foods at Nine to Ten Months 146
    Foods at Eleven to Twelve Months 146
Sample Meal Plan From Six to Twelve Months............................... 147
    Six Months 147
    Seven to Eight Months.. 147
    Nine to Ten Months 147
    Eleven to Twelve Months... 147
Nutritional Considerations 148

REFERENCES **151**

Introduction:

Welcome to Motherhood

Sometimes, being a mom feels like being born with superpowers. It's a significant duty, but also like going on a magical journey. You're now a member of the fantastic club called motherhood, whether you're a new mom or taking care of your second or third child. Your life turns into a fascinating story, like a fairy tale. Every day is a fresh start with lots of joy, happiness, and wonder. Having a baby isn't just having a baby; it's like making a drink full of love and happiness. The love of a mother is the only love that doesn't change. Mothers hold their children's hands and guide them through life's ups and downs. Every mother is always there for her kids, no matter what, to cheer them up and keep them going. For women, motherhood is a beautiful but dangerous and stressful time. Only pregnant women and moms can describe and understand a lot of the stress and pressure they're under. Things need to change when you become a mom—not because you want them to, but because they have to. Undoubtedly, it's one of the hardest things a woman can do.

Being pregnant makes your body feel like a secret garden full of things that could happen. It's like a tiny person is saying hello when you feel little flutters inside. The baby's kicks feel like high fives, and you feel like you have an incredible secret. In the quiet moments, you feel like you have a special bond with your baby. It's like talking to the stars in private. You're not just going to be a mom soon; you're going to be a fighter who protects dreams.

Postpartum women encounter various obstacles after giving birth, and it's important to remember that their job doesn't end there. The time after giving birth is a fantastic part of becoming a mother, and it comes with challenges and rewards. From getting better physically to riding the mental roller coaster, moms undergo significant changes that need time, understanding, and help. Self-care is no longer a nice to have. It's a must, and asking for help is a sign of strength, not weakness. There are changes, pressures, and enormous responsibilities that come with being a mom. If a woman isn't ready or has no help, these things can sometimes be too much for her. When a woman has to handle it alone, it can be not very comforting if it's not done right.

Hello, I'm Eliza Kindler, and I'm thrilled to embark on this journey with you through the pages of this book. As a mother of three little ones, my experience of motherhood is as unique as each of my children. My inspiration for this journey comes from the shared challenges my sister and I faced during the postpartum period, especially in the realm of getting our babies to latch for feeding. Her struggles mirrored my own, pushing me to explore the uncharted territories of the postpartum journey. Together, we navigated these challenges, prioritizing our health and seeking the support we needed. Initially, frustration loomed large when my daughter wouldn't latch, but through those early struggles, I learned a valuable lesson—using formula isn't a failure. It's a choice made with love and the well-being of our little ones in mind.

Join me as I unfold the pages of my story, sharing the highs, the lows, and the triumphs that come with being a mom navigating the beautiful chaos of motherhood. My main goal is to motivate new and experienced moms to care for themselves and prioritize their health while also being good moms. In *The No B.S. Guide to Postpartum Care*, I share unfiltered, practical advice for new moms, offering insights on physical recovery and emotional resilience after childbirth. I understand the chaos that follows birth and aim to provide a resource that speaks directly to postpartum needs. Combining professional knowledge with personal experience, I address misconceptions, offer recovery strategies, and support mothers in reclaiming their wellness amid the whirlwind of parenthood. My book is a movement toward a more honest and self-compassionate approach to the transformative journey of motherhood.

A child's view of the world is mainly based on how their mother sees it. Being a mother includes life's stages: goals, dreams, acceptance, mistakes, losses, turning away from sin, and forgiving. It shows how determined a mother is to prepare her child for the challenges that will come in life and to teach the next generation about the different ways to live. A mother's well-being is just as important as that of her child.

Therefore, she shouldn't neglect her needs or put her development behind her child's.

Finally, I want to stress how important it is for new moms to give themselves the time and room they need after giving birth. It's important to say no to the push to "bounce back" or "enjoy every minute" as being a mom can be tricky. Accept that healing takes time and enjoy the beauty of your unique path. Keep in mind that every step forward is a victory. Let go of any negative messages around you that make you have unreasonably high standards. You should instead be kind to yourself, enjoy the little wins, and know that it's okay to not have everything worked out. Being a mother changes you, and your health is the most important thing. So, moms, please be kind and patient with yourselves and let yourselves heal and grow at your own pace. You're doing a great job, and your journey is yours alone to enjoy.

Chapter 1:

Understanding the Fourth

Trimester

Everyone knows that the beautiful process of pregnancy has three distinct phases or trimesters. However, this story has a twist: Have you ever heard of the enigmatic and sometimes ignored "fourth trimester"? Postpartum is like this period's unacknowledged hero; it doesn't usually receive the recognition it deserves. So, the main issue is: Do you know what this fourth trimester is about and how it feels? Now is the time to fasten your seatbelts as we enter the unknown area of the fourth trimester, a period of changes, discoveries, and a great deal of love.

The time after giving birth, sometimes known as the fourth trimester, is critical for both the mother and the baby. During this time, the mother and infant must be close and linked on numerous levels. Do you know what "matrescence" means? It's like the maternal equivalent of a secret sauce; if you know it, the fourth trimester will make much more sense. When a woman becomes a mother, she experiences a dramatic change known as matrescence. The birth of a child brings about profound changes in a person's life, both physically and emotionally. It's like the birth of a new self, including the role of motherhood (Cradlewise Staff, 2023).

The Fourth Trimester

You will already know that the first, second, and third trimesters are different steps of pregnancy During these trimesters, your baby grows and changes while still in your belly. The fourth trimester is the three months (12 weeks) after giving birth. The term was first used in 2002 by American pediatrician Harvey Karp to emphasize that even if your baby is physically separate from you, you and your infant remain inseparable. In many ways, your baby is still developing and operating as if in utero; they entirely rely on you while transitioning to life outside the womb (*What to Expect in the Fourth Trimester*, n.d.).

It's crucial to remember that throughout a newborn's first few months, mom and baby have a biological need to be close. The infant has a physiological need for the mother's assistance, and both have an emotional desire to be near each other, touch, and take in each other's scents. By learning more about the science underpinning the postpartum period, we can better appreciate the role it plays in the maturation of the brain and neurological system. A mother's stress levels and how her nervous system reacts to the environment have a lasting impact on her child, just as they do throughout motherhood (*The 4th Trimester*, 2023).

The fourth trimester of pregnancy is a time of great intensity, and it may be difficult if you don't know what to anticipate. You're dealing with sleep deprivation on top of the typical and anticipated difficulties of recuperating from birth, processing your birth experience, learning to interpret your baby's signs, and establishing a nursing rhythm or feeding regimen. At the same time as the enormous hormonal changes you're experiencing, you enter a period of profound uncertainty.

Fourth Trimester for Babies

After nine months of being in your warm womb, your baby has to get used to many new sights, sounds, and smells, as well as a colder environment without your amniotic fluid to support them. In the first three months after being born, your baby will need much of your attention and affection. It might be difficult for them to adjust to the outside world after nine months of being protected from it in your womb. Your infant will seek solace in your arms, your voice, and your touch. It's more important to read your baby's signs and help them feel secure during this time than to stick to a strict schedule.

Babies in the womb are used to their mothers' constant care, which includes feeding, rocking, and sleep. After they are born, we add pauses between feedings and put them in a separate area to sleep. Understandably, they can find this terrifying; they are also expected to weep out of fear (National Childbirth Trust, 2023).

In a nutshell, the fourth trimester is a period of intense connection, focusing on responsiveness and caring. As you and your baby go through this beautiful change together, you can look forward to many opportunities to connect, share hugs and kisses, and provide care around the clock.

Physical Changes

The fourth trimester is a time of fantastic growth and change for moms. Your body goes through several remarkable transformations during the postpartum period. In addition to the physical changes that lead to postpartum recovery, mothers also experience profound psychological and hormonal upheavals:

- **Healing and recovery:** Your body did something unique, so prepare for the healing process. Whether you gave birth vaginally or via a C-section, your body is still working hard to heal. As your body heals, you may feel sore, have stitches, and always be tired.

- **Repair reproductive organs:** There will be stitches and pain during the healing process for women who tore during delivery. Sitz baths, witch hazel pads, and soothing sprays can help you feel better after giving birth. Also, don't forget how important rest is—your body needs it to heal.

- **Perineal pain:** It is expected to experience pain in the perineum, especially after a surgical procedure or tears. A donut cushion, warm clothes, and good hygiene can help. It's essential to keep the area clean to avoid illness.

- **Hormonal changes:** Hormones are like the directors of this postpartum concert. Changes in them can cause mood swings, emotional highs and lows, and even tears. It's normal to feel a lot of different emotions at this point.

- **Changes in the breasts:** If you decide to breastfeed your infant, your breasts will change. As your milk supply changes to meet your baby's needs, they may get full, sore, or swollen. Finding a nursing bra that fits well and supports your breasts can make all the difference.

- **Nipple pain:** Although breastfeeding is a lovely part of the bonding process, it may be difficult. A painful nipple can be alleviated with the proper latch, lanolin lotion, and air time. A lactation consultant's advice may be helpful.

- **Changes in hair and skin:** Your hair and skin may change because of hormone changes. While some women lose their hair, others notice changes in their skin, such as acne or spots getting darker or lighter. Note that these changes will only last for a short time and are typically caused by hormones.

- **Uterine contractions:** Your uterus is now contracting back to its prepregnancy size. It has grown to make room for your growing baby. These contractions, sometimes called "afterpains," can be felt more strongly when nursing.

- **Postpartum bleeding:** Postpartum bleeding, sometimes called lochia, occurs when the uterine lining is lost after giving birth. It's like menstruation, except the bleeding may be thicker initially. The rate of discharge progressively decreases as time progresses.

- **Pain in the joints and muscles:** Pregnancy and childbirth are hard on your body. Pain and discomfort are possible, particularly in the hips and lower back. Light stretching and exercise help ease aches and pains.

- **Pre-eclampsia:** Pre-eclampsia is a severe medical condition characterized by dangerously high blood pressure in a pregnant woman. After giving birth, it's essential to keep an eye out for things like headaches, eyesight problems, and stomach discomfort.

- **Heavy bleeding:** When symptoms like soaking through pads continue, it's a sign of heavy bleeding, which is a severe medical condition that may occur after childbirth (Catholic Health Initiatives, n.d.).

Because every woman is different, these changes may not happen to everyone. However, you can make the transition to the fourth trimester easier by taking things one day at a time, getting help, and prioritizing yourself.

Emotions and Mental Health

When a baby is born, mothers can feel many strong feelings, from joy and excitement to fear and worry. But it can also lead to depression, which is not what you might expect. However, this is a significant time for both moms and babies as they deal with the physical and mental changes that arise after giving birth. The mental health of both the mother and the baby need to be understood.

Let me tell you about my postpartum journey with my firstborn, which didn't start easily. My labor went on for more than 30 hours, and it ended with an emergency cesarean section. The next day, as I was trying to breastfeed, I faced a challenge—my baby had trouble latching, and she was crying a lot. The nurse suggested switching to formula for a few days to ease the situation.

I found it hard to put my emotions into words. I describe it as an overwhelming and disconnected feeling, like floating above my body, watching everything unfold without understanding it.

I experienced unexpected bursts of emotions, felt alone, and was filled with anxiety. I recalled sitting beside my daughter on my bed, watching my husband drive away for work. I felt I didn't want to be alone because

I was afraid that I might not know what to do or mess things up. I felt a sudden panic, with irrational thoughts racing through my mind.

It was a challenging time for me, but sharing these experiences can help others understand the emotional roller coaster that some new mothers go through. To best care for new mothers, it is vital to understand the dramatic dynamic changes inside the body after giving birth.

Emotional Aspects for Moms

- **Changes in hormones:** Changes in levels of hormones like estrogen and progesterone happen after giving birth. Changes in hormones can make you irritable, have mood swings, and feel sad, also known as the "baby blues." The baby blues are a mild form of sadness that only lasts for a short time. Once the hormones level out, the baby blues go away. Almost all new moms—up to 85% of them—will feel down after giving birth. One minute, you might be happy, and the next, you might be upset and cry. "No mother is ever happy. It's okay to get angry and even need to put the baby down sometimes" (Johns Hopkins Medicine, n.d.). Those who have a history of anxiety, depression, or bipolar illness have a 30–35% increased risk of developing postpartum depression (PPD). Also, moms who had symptoms of depression after prior pregnancies are more likely to have them following their subsequent pregnancies (Johns Hopkins Medicine, n.d.).

- **PPD:** Some women may have worse mood conditions that last longer, like PPD. People with PPD may feel very sad, depressed, tired, and like they're not good enough. Family and loved ones need to know the signs and be there to help. Depression after childbirth may last for months or even years if not treated. In one study, 25% of participants were still feeling sadness three years after the birth of their infants. That's why getting checked out and seeking treatment immediately is crucial (Johns Hopkins Medicine, n.d.).

- **Body image issues:** After giving birth, many women notice changes in their bodies, which can make them feel bad about their self-esteem. The body needs time to heal, and social pressure to "bounce back" quickly can make people feel like they're not good enough. It is often believed that women should be able to "bounce back" to their prepregnancy state quickly after giving birth. This misconception may be fostered by "cultural norms" shown by celebrities who return to the spotlight soon after giving birth, seemingly unfazed by the myriad of adjustments necessary to care for a newborn. These assumptions could not be further from reality, and shattering these unreasonable expectations is vital to enabling a woman to bask in parenthood's normality. A woman's body needs one to two years to heal after being pregnant and giving birth, but this is not what women are taught to think. Think about the good things your body has done and the wonder it has made as a new mother instead of the things you might not like about it or the things you wish were different (Karges, 2023).

- **Lack of sleep:** New moms often have trouble getting enough sleep, which can heighten emotional reactions. Researchers say that changes in the body and mind during and after birth may worsen sleeplessness. A recent study in Spain looked at 486 pregnant women to see if they had insomnia and found that over 33% complained of severe insomnia (Iavarone, 2023).

- **Role change:** Becoming a mother dramatically alters your personality and roles. Some mothers find it challenging to adjust to their new role, which can lead to stress and mental problems.

Emotional Aspects for Babies

- **Bonding and attachment:** Establishing a secure attachment in the first few weeks after birth is essential for bonding and development. Attachment is strengthened by loving relationships and care given and received with open hearts (*Attachment: A Connection for Life*, n.d.).

- **Feeding challenges:** Problems with feeding can be emotionally draining for both the mother and the infant, whether they arise from breastfeeding difficulties or anxieties about switching to formula. Successfully overcoming these challenges requires help and advice. It's a common misconception that infants are born already knowing how to latch on and adequately nurse. Finding the proper latch takes a lot of time, a lot of practice, and, yes, some sore nipples. A baby taking the nipple and areola of their mother's breast into their mouth to feed is called "latching on." It is, without a doubt, the most significant component of the breastfeeding process. Your baby will not be able to obtain the milk they need, and your breasts will not be encouraged to create more milk, which will start a vicious cycle of low milk demand and low milk supply. If your baby does not have the correct latch, they will not get the milk they require (O'Connor, 2022).

- **Sensory overload:** Because babies are so open to their environment, they may experience sensory overload. A soothing and comforting atmosphere may significantly improve your newborn's mental health.

- **Developmental milestones:** Babies experience many changes in the first few months of life. It is crucial to be sensitive to their needs and provide a stimulating environment during each stage of development.

The above information acknowledges the relationships among postpartum physical, emotional, and mental wellness. It stresses the need to receive professional care for depression and anxiety since a mother's mental health affects bonding, confidence, and newborn development.

Common Challenges

We've already talked about the problems women can have after giving birth. However, many women have a smooth return after pregnancy, labor, and delivery. There are, however, problems that can happen after the baby is born. The following are some of the most usual challenges:

- sleep deprivation

- breast and breastfeeding problems, breast pain, and tenderness such as swollen breasts, clogged milk ducts, or mastitis

- digestive issues and colorectal problems such as incontinence (both urinary and fecal), constipation, and hemorrhoids

- hair loss

- vaginal pain

- backache

- perineal pain after birth (the perineum is the area between the vaginal opening and the anus)

- if a C-section was done, pain at the scar site

- pain or discomfort during sex

- vaginal discharge

- stretch marks

Navigating the postpartum period takes awareness, resilience, and a willingness to seek help (*Potential Postpartum Problems*, n.d.).

Feeling any of these feelings is expected. It's also okay to feel different every day or minute. Supporting new moms to care for themselves and learn how to care for their babies is very important.

Chapter 2:

Physical Recovery After Childbirth

As mothers, we are likely overjoyed to be home with our new baby after nine months of waiting. It's possible that your baby's birth was complicated or simple. You may have had a vaginal birth or a cesarean birth (C-section). It's possible that you worked hard for hours or days. No matter what your birth looked like, your body has been through a lot; it will need some time to get better. Giving birth is hard on the body, and the time afterward is crucial for healing. When a woman gives birth, her body usually changes during labor. Her muscles, joints, and organs need time to heal. C-sections, meanwhile, involve surgery on the abdomen, which makes the healing process more difficult. Regardless of the mode of birth, both entail hormone changes and a slow return to full physical strength.

This chapter describes how to care for your body during this crucial time. This is because healing after giving birth has its own set of problems. This chapter gives moms useful information to help them deal with the physical parts of life after giving birth. It also talks about how important rest is for healing. It offers many tools to help create a loving space for healing and having a good time after giving birth.

After Delivery

The time right after giving birth is significant for both the baby and the parents. For a better transition into life after giving birth, knowing what to expect during this time is essential. You won't be fully recovered in just a few days; postpartum recovery can take months. Many women feel mostly better after six to eight weeks, but it could take longer than that to feel like yourself again. You might feel like your body has turned against you at this point. Do your best not to get angry. Keep in mind that your physical self is unaware of your goals and deadlines. Resting, eating well, and taking breaks are the best things you can do for it. Your body spends months getting ready for birth, and it takes time to heal afterward. It might take even longer if you've had a cesarean, since it takes longer to heal from surgery. If the C-section was unanticipated, it may have also caused some emotional problems (*Recovering From Delivery*, 2023).

What to Expect

In the early stages of healing after giving birth, it's essential to move slowly and gently. Here are some of the things you can expect.

Body Aches

Muscle stiffness and general exhaustion are common side effects of intense physical labor and delivery. Muscle and joint pain may be exacerbated by hormonal changes, such as decreased estrogen and progesterone after delivery. Some women have abdominal pains and flutters (similar to menstruation cramps) as their uterus shrinks back to its prepregnancy size, and these symptoms often worsen while nursing. Body pains may be a symptom of the general exhaustion brought on by the responsibilities of caring for a baby, including frequent feedings and disturbed sleep patterns. If you've had an episiotomy or a cesarean section, the healing process might create localized discomfort and contribute to total body stiffness. A lack of proper water and nourishment may worsen muscular weariness, aches, and pains. However, prescribed or over-the-counter pain medication should alleviate the problem within a few days.

Swollen Feet and Extremities

Fluid retention is common throughout pregnancy. It may take some time for your body to regain its natural fluid balance and expel any extra fluids after giving birth, particularly if IV fluids were used during labor. Swelling of the hands, cheeks, ankles, neck, and other extremities (edema) may be caused by hormonal shifts. In fact, it's typical for your feet to grow by half a size. Elimination of the surplus fluids may take many weeks. To hasten the process, choose foods rich in potassium, such as vegetables and fruits—this helps counteract the water-retaining effects of sodium—and drink more than the suggested eight glasses of water per day, particularly if you are breastfeeding.

To manage swollen feet and extremities after delivery

- elevate your feet

- stay hydrated

- move regularly

- avoid salty foods

- wear compression socks to reduce swelling

Enlarged Breasts

A lot of moms find that for the first day or two after giving birth, their breasts get red, swollen, painful, and full of milk. After the swelling goes down, your breasts will likely start to sag after three to four days or until you stop nursing. This is because the skin will be too tight. You may also leak milk for a few weeks, even if you don't breastfeed your baby. You may also notice that the nipple looks off. Postpartum breast engorgement or enlargement is normal, but it can be painful. If you are not nursing or pumping, you can help ease the discomfort by wearing a supportive bra and using cold compresses to reduce pain and swelling.

Urinary Incontinence

Many women have urinary incontinence after giving birth, although this is usually short-lived. Weakened or injured pelvic floor muscles as a result of the pressure imposed on them during pregnancy and birth can contribute to urinary incontinence. Two main types of urine leakage can happen after giving birth:

- **Incontinence due to stress:** When you cough, sneeze, laugh, or lift something heavy, you might leak pee. This is an example of this type of accidental leakage.

- **Urge incontinence:** This type, which is also called overactive bladder, causes a quick, strong need to go to the bathroom, which often makes it impossible to get there in time.

See a doctor if urine leakage persists or causes trouble. They can give you a personalized evaluation, help you with exercises, and suggest the best ways to address the underlying causes of your leakage.

Varicose Veins

During and after childbirth, many women get varicose veins. This is usually because of extra pressure on the blood vessels in the pelvic and lower body areas. Up to 40% of pregnant women get swollen blood vessels near the skin's surface, most often on the calves and thighs. Genetics, hormones, and the extra weight that puts pressure on the veins during pregnancy all play a part. The condition is usually only temporary, and varicose veins may get better after giving birth, but they can take up to 12 weeks to go away (Brown-Worsham, 2023).

Self-Care

We've already talked about the most common problems that women face after giving birth, such as not getting enough sleep, vaginal bleeding, and bladder problems. Next, we will talk about strategic self-care steps you can take to avoid getting infections and speed up your healing. These methods will give you all the information you need for a healthy and happy postpartum period.

After a Cesarean

Women who have had a cesarean section need to pay special attention to the incision region and ensure adequate abdominal support. After using the restroom, rinse the incision area with warm water from a peri bottle and wipe it dry with a clean towel to prevent inflammation. Wear loose, comfortable clothes and an abdominal binder or maternity belt to help support your pooch if your doctor recommends it. Walking or light exercise should be introduced gradually to improve circulation and lessen stiffness. Reducing muscular pain using a heating pad set to a low setting and taking prescription pain medication may aid in a speedier recovery.

After a Vaginal Birth

Perineal care is of the utmost importance for moms who have given birth vaginally. Use a peri bottle filled with warm water for post-toilet washing, and ensure that the perineal region is dried with a clean towel as soon as possible after using the bathroom to avoid irritation. Choose postpartum underwear made of mesh or use the ones supplied by the hospital. Cotton underwear that is breathable and does not apply pressure should be your first choice. If you are experiencing discomfort in the perineal region, sitz baths may give calming relief; nevertheless, it is essential to speak with your healthcare professional before using them. Start doing pelvic floor exercises (Kegels) gradually to build up your pelvic muscles. Pain management strategies that improve overall comfort include taking prescribed pain medicines and applying a cold compress to minimize swelling.

Pain Management

Pain is a frequent element of the journey that expectant moms face as part of the unique difficulties of the postpartum period. Women's perceptions of pain vary greatly, regardless of whether they are anticipating a cesarean section or a vaginal delivery. Realizing that every delivery is unique, moms must take measures to alleviate their discomfort before it gets unbearable. Alternative treatments like acupuncture and physical therapy might give extra assistance in addition to the recommended drug alternatives offered by healthcare experts. Hot or cold treatment and herbal supplements are examples of natural therapies that may be used as an adjunct to conventional pain medication. Providing women with various pain management strategies boosts their confidence and makes them feel more in charge of their health and happiness at this extraordinary time. Let's talk about postpartum pain management now.

Medication Options

- **Prescription painkillers:** If you're having pain after giving birth, especially if you had a cesarean section, your doctor may recommend painkillers. Take them as advised to get good pain relief.

- **Over-the-counter pain relievers:** If you have your healthcare provider's permission, pain relievers like acetaminophen or ibuprofen can ease light to moderate postpartum pain.

Painkillers that your doctor or nurse prescribes are safe to take while nursing, and you should follow the directions to stay relaxed. Get as much rest as possible, and don't lift anything heavier than your baby (*Postpartum Pain Management*, n.d.).

Alternative Therapies

In addition to medical care, alternative therapies are used to heal the mind, the body, or both. Before you start any alternative treatments, especially while you are pregnant or right after giving birth, talk to your doctor. Alternative treatments shouldn't be used instead of crucial medicine. Some therapies are not part of the regular medical care that doctors usually recommend; these are called complementary therapies. Acupuncture, massage, and naturopathy are different types of alternative treatments. They're also sometimes known as "integrative medicine."

Other than supplemental therapies, which are used *alongside* regular medical care from your doctor, alternative therapies are used *instead of* such care. Pregnant women may utilize alternative treatments to decrease nausea and back discomfort. These treatments may also help women prepare for labor and have a smooth birth. Postpartum, these approaches assist mothers in doing physical exercises to strengthen muscles, improve posture, and relieve back and pelvic discomfort. Now, let's discuss the different types of alternative therapies that help postpartum.

Chiropractic and Osteopathy

- The goal of these treatments is to ease low-back and pelvic pain, which is widespread during and after pregnancy.

- It's unclear how well they work, but they are usually considered safe for pregnant women and those who have recently given birth. These treatments can help adjust the spine and hips after birth, easing pain and improving general joint health.

Massage

- Pregnancy massage aims to help women cope with their changing bodies, lower their stress, and sleep better.

- As far as effectiveness goes, it relaxes you and eases muscle strain.

- Massage can also help after giving birth, relieving lingering stress, encouraging relaxation, and easing the pain and soreness of the muscles used during labor.

Reflexology

- Reflexology aims to ease pain in the lower back or pelvis by stimulating certain parts of the feet.

- It is said to be safe and may help with pain.

- Reflexology can help with hip or lower back pain that doesn't go away after giving birth, making you feel better and more relaxed.

Naturopathy

- Naturopathy promotes health through natural methods, such as a healthy diet, plant medicines, and regular exercise.

- There is little research on this, but the method is generally broad and focuses on supporting overall health.

- Nutrition and plant supplements can be significant components of naturopathic treatments for new mothers, helping them heal and feel better.

Hypnotherapy

- Hypnosis is used to ease the pain of birth and lower stress.

- It takes time, but it can help during labor.

- Hypnotherapy methods can also be used to help new moms deal with stress after giving birth by assisting them to relax and calm down.

Biofeedback Training

- Biofeedback is used to help women understand and control their body's childbirth indicators.

- There is a limited amount of high-quality data, but the goal is to make people more aware of their body's reactions.

- It's not clear if biofeedback training can help ease labor pain, but it can make you more aware of how your body is reacting after giving birth, which can help you relax and deal with stress.

When new moms consider alternative treatments, they should talk to their doctors to ensure they are safe and suitable for their postpartum situation (Healthdirect Australia, n.d.-b).

Natural Remedies

As a new mother, your mind and body are going through tremendous changes. Before you go through the postpartum stage, I think you should give it some thought. This can provide you with time to get a few natural remedies that will help you feel better after giving birth, which should make your transition to being a mom a little easier. Perineal pain, after-pains, and mood changes after giving birth are all regular problems that women face. Many women have pain in their vagina, vulva, and perineal area after giving birth. Urinating can often make you feel some stinging. A perineal bottle can help ease this while going to the bathroom. A spray bottle full of herbs can also help a lot. For the first few days, some women like to go to the bathroom in a sitz bath.

My favorite plants to care for the perineum are lavender, marigold, rose, comfrey, sage, yarrow, and Himalayan salt. You can make these as if making strong tea and then put them in a spray bottle to clean up after going to the bathroom. They are very relaxing and help your body heal. You can also add witch hazel to your list of natural medicines after giving birth. It can be put on pads to make them feel better. To help lower pain and swelling, it's also important to rest as much as possible. You can also use other remedies, like applying hot and cold compresses to affected areas. Warmth can soothe muscle soreness, while cold can reduce swelling and numb pain.

Specific herbal remedies, such as arnica or witch hazel, may provide relief. Always consult with a healthcare provider before using herbal supplements. Safe essential oils like lavender or chamomile used in aromatherapy can help you relax and feel less pain. Ensure you dilute the oils correctly and talk to a professional (Stewart, 2018).

Practical Tips for Overall Pain Management

- **Hydration:** Staying hydrated helps your body heal and can ease headaches and sore muscles.

- **Balanced nutrition:** To help your body heal and stay healthy, eat a balanced diet full of nutrients.

- **Adequate rest:** Make rest a priority and get enough sleep to help your body heal.

Exercises and Stretches

Becoming a mother brings about profound changes in a woman's life, affecting various aspects from daily routines to overall lifestyle. Let's talk about your workout routine!

How soon after giving birth can you start working out again? Pay attention to your body. The best time for each person to start moving again after giving birth depends on things like the type of birth they had, their general health, and any problems they had during labor. However, you shouldn't do hard or strenuous workouts until after your postpartum checkup, which is usually around six weeks after giving birth.

The time after giving birth is crucial and needs a slow and gentle approach to exercise. It will help if you do gentle movements and stretches while healing to develop strength, especially in your pelvic floor and core muscles. These routines not only help you get back to being physically healthy, but they also help you recover after giving birth and get back to being functionally fit. Your stomach and pelvic floor muscles get weaker during pregnancy and childbirth. This is significant because these muscle groups contribute to stability and balance in everyday life and during physical activity. Following pregnancy, it is essential to restore muscular strength in these areas, and engaging in postpartum exercises is an effective means to achieve this objective.

A safe workout plan for after giving birth can include the following.

Pelvic Floor Strengthening Exercises

Kegel Exercises

- **Goal:** Make the muscles in the pelvic floor stronger.

- **Steps:** Lift and squeeze the pelvic floor muscles as if you were stopping the flow of pee. Hold for a short time, then let go.

- **Caution:** Make sure your bladder is empty before starting this exercise, and don't press down on or squeeze your bottom.

Pelvic Tilts

- **Goal:** Strengthen the hip muscles and the lower back.

- **Steps:** Lie on your back with your knees bent. Pull your abs in and slowly lift your hips off the ground. Then, slowly lower them.

- **Caution:** If you have diastasis recti (see below), be careful and don't arch your back too much.

Core Strengthening Exercises

Heel Slides

- **Goal:** Work out your abs and keep your core tight.

- **Steps:** Lie on your back with your knees bent. Slide one heel along the floor to straighten the leg and return it to its original position.

- **Caution:** Keep your lower back pressed into the floor and do the move slowly.

Seated Leg Lifts

- **Goal:** Make the muscles in your lower abdomen stronger.

- **Steps:** Sit on the edge of a chair with your back straight. Lift one leg straight out in front of you. Hold for a few seconds, then bring it back down.

- **Caution:** Keep your back straight, and don't lean back.

Overall Well-Being Exercises

Deep Breathing Exercises

- **Goal:** Help you relax and engage your core.

- **Steps:** Take a deep breath, which will widen your diaphragm, and exhale completely, tightening your abdominal muscles.

- **Caution:** To avoid stressing, focus on taking slow, easy breaths.

Cat/Cow Yoga Stretches

- **Goal:** Move the spine, stretch the back, and work the core.

- **Steps:** Begin by getting down on your knees and hands. Breathe in as you arch your back (cow), and breathe out as you round your spine (cat).

- **Caution:** Move slowly, and don't bend your back too far or squeeze your lower back too hard.

After giving birth, you should be very careful about the types of abdominal and pelvic muscle exercises you do. Returning to high-intensity core workouts too quickly will aggravate your weakened abdominal and pelvic muscles (McCallum, 2021).

Postpartum Recovery Tips

- Start your workouts slowly and pay attention to what your body is telling you.

- Talk to your doctor before starting any workout plan, especially if you have problems during labor or birth.

- One in two pregnant women have diastasis recti, or two separated abs, after giving birth (De Bellefonds, 2023). Diastasis recti is a health condition where the distance between your rectus abdominis muscles (also known as a "six-pack") grows across the midline. This happens because the connective tissue (linea alba) stretches, making the muscles feel less stable and causing the abdomen to bulge or constrict. Some women may look like they are "still pregnant" because they have this condition, which raises the pressure inside the abdomen. It's also known as "mummy tummy" or "mommy pouch." Please pay attention to your diastasis recti and avoid workouts that worsen it.

- The connective tissue gets weaker and thinner when belly fat pushes through it or the uterus grows and puts pressure on it. Giving birth can also change the pressure inside the abdomen in many ways. Because of pregnancy hormones and the growing uterus, the weight of the fetus is pushed down to the pelvis, which can cause diastasis recti. Because of this, you should avoid any exercise that makes your stomach stick out or heavy lifting exercises that require you to twist or extend your spine (Shiraz, 2022).

- Maintaining a healthy diet and enough fluid intake will aid in the healing process.

These exercises are intended to aid in the early stages of recovery. Focus on slow, gentle motions and make any necessary adjustments based on how your body responds. Always speak with healthcare specialists for specialized advice and assistance.

Rest and Self-Care

New moms must take time for relaxation and self-care in the chaos of caring for a baby. Getting adequate sleep during this time might be difficult, but it's essential for a mom's physical and mental health while she adjusts to parenting. The difficulties encountered by mothers at this time include

- crying

- irritability

- insomnia

- sadness

- mood swings

- restlessness

After giving birth, it is expected to have emotional ups and downs. During the postpartum period, the baby blues affect over 80% of new mothers (*Postpartum Care for Mom*, n.d.). To overcome this, we need to practice self-care, such as

- getting as much sleep as possible

- embracing the support of those close to you

- engaging in your relationship by spending time with your partner

- starting a workout routine

- following your physician's advice (*Postpartum Care for Mom*, n.d.)

Self-Care Practices for Physical Well-Being

- **Relaxation techniques:** Postpartum relaxation practices provide physical and mental assistance for new moms. Physical healing, hormonal changes, and baby care may make the postpartum period difficult. Practicing relaxation methods every day helps provide calm, decrease tension, and improve well-being. Deep breathing, meditation, yoga, aromatherapy, warm baths, and more are used. Mothers should learn to unwind by delving into deep breathing exercises and other relaxation techniques.

- **Mindfulness exercises:** Meditation and light yoga are great ways to develop mindfulness and bring calmness and focus into your life.

- **Pampering routines:** Rejuvenate your body and mind with self-care routines like taking a long, hot shower, getting a massage, or treating yourself to a luxurious facial.

Don't be stressed out. Enjoy every moment of quiet time with your baby. It may take some time to feel like your usual self again. We will discuss this topic in more detail in Chapter 9, which is a complete resource for maternal self-care and well-being. We will examine various practices and ways to support your physical and mental well-being throughout the postpartum journey, with more tailored recommendations and instructions for navigating the postpartum period.

Warning Signs

Mothers must be checked up after giving birth because of the possibility of significant and perhaps fatal complications. Inadequate postpartum care results in the early demise of far too many mothers.

How do you know if something is just a natural part of getting well, or if you should be worried? A lot of moms have the same worries. Talking to doctors and nurses is an effective way to ensure your health and deal with any worries you might have during this time.

As you will be focused on caring for a newborn, you may overlook the early warning signs of your own health issues. Pay attention to the indicators below that suggest something might be wrong and may point to particular health concerns:

- excessive or prolonged pain in the abdomen, perineum, or incision site

- vaginal bleeding that lasts longer than the average time after giving birth

- fever or chills that don't go away, which could be a sign of an infection

- foul-smelling vaginal discharge

- signs of deep vein thrombosis; your legs may be red, swollen, or sore

- having trouble breathing

- persistent headaches or changes in vision

- urinary or bowel issues

- notable mood swings

- appearance of new lumps, bumps, or sore spots, especially in the breasts (*Warning Signs of Postpartum Health Problems*, n.d.)

It's important to remember that everyone recovers differently and that some pain or changes is expected after giving birth. But you must see a doctor immediately if you have any warning signs or other symptoms that make you nervous. Early help can prevent problems and ensure safer and more effective healing.

Chapter 3:

Emotional Well-Being and Mental

Health

After having a baby, some women may feel a little unhappy if things don't go as anticipated during labor. Women who planned for a vaginal birth but had to have an emergency C-section are more vulnerable to these feelings, especially if this is their first child. C-section mothers may have feelings of shame or disappointment when they hear positive remarks about vaginal birth from others. While some mothers may regret their decision to undergo a cesarean section, others may not. You can feel like you didn't do things "properly" or that you lost control if the birth didn't go as planned. You might even feel guilty for "failing" your child. You can feel as if you lost out on something by having to receive general anesthesia for the C-section. Although hearing the opinions of others might be frustrating, remember that you know your child and yourself best. It might be helpful to talk to other parents who have had C-sections. Having been there themselves, they may provide insight into how to deal with unhelpful feedback. Though it may be challenging right now, these emotions will pass. The most important thing is that you and your baby are healthy and safe, since every mother's experience is different.

It's not easy when people around you oppose you, or you're feeling low. Instead of letting your emotions rule you, get help regulating them and reach out for assistance. Talking to someone you trust or getting expert guidance can make a huge difference. Remember that you can get help to work through your emotions and that others care about you and want to help you. Taking charge of your emotional state and reaching out for help are potent strategies for facing adversity and finding your footing again.

Emotional well-being is strongly linked to mental health. Mothers can handle the emotional ups and downs that come with hormonal changes, not getting enough sleep, and taking on new tasks like caring for a baby if they have good mental health. A mentally healthy mother is more likely to respond to and care for her child, which builds a strong emotional bond between them. Having good mental health makes it easier for a mother to make decisions and deal with stress. It gives her the strength and flexibility to deal with problems that come out of the blue and make intelligent decisions for herself and her baby.

As we talked about in Chapter 1, the time after giving birth is marked by significant changes in hormones that can affect a new mom's mental health. These changes, along with getting used to life with a baby, make many moms feel a lot of different feelings. People often feel sad during this time, called the "baby blues."

Understanding the Baby Blues

The months after the birth of a child can be beautiful but challenging for both parents and others in the household. These first few weeks after giving birth are rife with novelty, emotional ups and downs, and, for some mothers, PPD. The "baby blues" are the unexpected sensations of sadness, irritation, crying, and restlessness that many new mothers report experiencing in the days and weeks after giving birth.

Having a baby is intended to make you joyful, not unhappy. Therefore, a depressed state of mind after giving birth might come as a shock to new mothers. Have hope: Although the baby blues aren't enjoyable, they usually don't last long, so you'll be back to normal (and smiling at your baby!) before you know it.

The postpartum blues often begin on day two or three and linger for many days or weeks. But there's good news: The baby blues generally go away independently, without any particular therapy, intervention, or medicine. Tell your doctor if you've been feeling down for over two weeks. They may want to see whether you have signs of PPD, a more severe disorder. PPD has symptoms in common with the "baby blues," but they are more intense and last for far longer.

Why Do New Mothers Feel So Down?

The postpartum blues might be the result of hormonal shifts. Mood swings are common after giving birth because estrogen and progesterone levels drop rapidly. Some people's thyroid glands produce much lower levels of hormones than usual, which may lead to extreme fatigue and mood swings. Not getting enough sleep and not eating adequately might contribute to these symptoms. Emotional difficulties are another probable cause of the baby blues. You may feel anxious about caring for your newborn or concerned about how your life has changed after birth. Sadness or depression may set in as a result of thinking such things.

If you've struggled with depression before, during, or after a previous pregnancy, you may be more likely to have PPD following the birth of your child.

Could Your Partner Have the Baby Blues?

Yes: 10% or more of partners may feel sad or depressed after the birth of a child. Sometimes, it starts up to a year after birth, but most of the time, it happens in the first three to six months (*Baby Blues After Pregnancy*, n.d.). Your spouse may be experiencing the baby blues if they

- withdraw and seek out isolation

- have mood swings, irritability, and nervousness

- lose interest in their job or favorite leisure activity, or decide to work more

- get down and out

- feel discouraged and overburdened

- struggle to fall asleep or make a choice

Depression can also be caused by not getting enough sleep, relationship issues, or stress. Hormones change during and after the birth of a baby, which can also make the father feel down. In new dads, testosterone levels may go down and estrogen levels may go up. Levels of many other chemicals, like cortisol, vasopressin, and prolactin, may increase. Every one of these changes in hormones can lead to sadness (*Baby Blues After Pregnancy*, n.d.).

Coping Strategies

Getting through the baby blues means using coping skills to make the mental change easier. One important thing is to ask family and friends for help. Talking about how you feel can help you feel better and give you confidence. Try the following:

- Communicate with loved ones.

- Rest.

- Accept help.

- Connect with other moms.

- Practice self-care.

Knowing that the baby blues are a common and short-term part of being a new mom can give mothers-to-be the strength to get through this stressful time with support and resolve.

Identifying and Managing PPD

Sad thoughts happen to everyone occasionally but generally go away in a few days. Depression gets in the way of daily life and can last for weeks or months at a time. With help, most people can get better, even those with the worst symptoms. PPD is a sadness that happens after giving birth. When you have PPD, your feelings are more potent and last longer than when you have the "baby blues." PPD is an actual mental illness that affects up to 25% of moms (Thompson, 2023). It's a lot worse than "the baby blues," which is mild sadness after giving birth. Several things help doctors figure out if someone has PPD:

- the signs

- the risk factors

- the differences from other mental illnesses

- the role of changes in hormone levels

Medical workers can help moms figure out how to deal with these issues so they can learn more about their mental health.

Recognizing Signs and Symptoms

- **Feeling sad or hopeless all the time:** A common sign of PPD is a chronic sadness or hopelessness that lasts longer than the first few weeks after giving birth. Mothers with PPD may find it hard to get rid of these intense feelings, which can make it hard for them to go about their daily lives.

- **Lost pleasure or interest:** Another common sign of PPD is an apparent loss of interest in things that used to be enjoyable. Some mothers lose interest in hobbies, social events, and other activities.

- **Sleep pattern changes:** PPD can disrupt a woman's regular sleep habits, causing her to have trouble sleeping or to sleep too much. These problems are worse than the usual sleep problems that come with caring for a baby and they have a significant effect on the mother's general health.

- **Changes in appetite:** PPD may be present if there are significant changes in hunger, such as an apparent rise or fall in appetite. These changes aren't just because of the work of parenting or caring for a newborn.

- **Muscular irritability or anger:** Mothers with PPD may feel irritable or angry, or have mood swings that are worse than the typical emotional problems that come with being a new mom. These feelings might not be in line with what's going on.

- **Feeling tired or losing energy all the time:** People with PPD often feel tired all the time and lose their energy. Mothers may constantly feel tired, making it hard to do daily chores or enjoy activities.

- **Having trouble focusing:** People with PPD may have trouble focusing, making choices, or clearing their minds, which can be called "mental fog." It can be challenging for them to concentrate on chores or remember things.

- **Health issues:** Physical symptoms that can't be explained, like headaches, stomachaches, or other aches and pains, may happen alongside PPD. Physical stresses don't just cause these symptoms; they're also connected to the mental problems that come with PPD.

- **Withdrawal from family and friends:** A lot of women who are going through PPD pull away from their family and friends, avoid social situations, and feel alone. Feelings of being cut off from others may make their general health worse.

- **Disturbing Ideas:** Thoughts of self-doubt, guilt, or hurting oneself or the baby may come to mothers with PPD and make it hard to concentrate. These thoughts can be upsetting and must be dealt with immediately by a professional.

Recognizing these symptoms and signs is essential for identifying problems quickly and getting help. If someone shows these signs, they need professional help immediately. PPD can be treated and, with the right help, moms can get through this challenging time and on their way to healing and well-being (Centers for Disease Control and Prevention, n.d.-b).

Strategies for Managing PPD

PPD needs to be treated in a way that takes into account both the mental and physical needs of the mother. Here are some of the strategies:

- Seek professional help from a therapist.

- Build a support system.

- Prioritize self-care.

- Explore medication and therapy.

- Create a routine.

- Set realistic goals.

- Connect with nature.

- Educate yourself.

- Monitor and reflect.

- Encourage open communication with your partner.

- Eat healthy and stay hydrated (Kinghorn, 2023).

Keep in mind that there may be some trial and error involved in finding the best approach to manage PPD. Getting the perfect mix of tactics might take time since everyone has a different story to tell. Be patient with yourself and remain dedicated to the road to recovery. The two most effective ways to recover from PPD are to get therapy and work on yourself.

PPD Self-Assessment Quiz

With all the changes and adjustments that parenting entails, it's essential to take care of your mental health. I've created this self-test to help you consider how the stress of caring for a new baby can affect your emotional well-being.

This test aims to help you assess how you've been feeling during the previous two weeks by considering factors such as mindset, sleep, physical health, and psychological health. By completing this self-assessment, you may learn more about your mental health and better understand the magnitude of your problems.

The self-assessment quiz has a scoring system that you can use to look for signs of PPD. Participants can choose to describe their events over a specific period. Please keep in mind that this quiz is not a medical tool. For a full review, people should get help from a professional.

Instructions

For each question, choose the answer that best describes your experiences in the last two weeks.

Question 1

Over the past two weeks, how often have you felt persistently sad or hopeless?

- 0: Not at all

- 1: Occasionally

- 2: Frequently

- 3: Most of the time

Question 2

In the last two weeks, how often have you lost interest or pleasure in activities you usually enjoy?

- 0: Not at all

- 1: Occasionally

- 2: Frequently

- 3: Most of the time

Question 3

Have you experienced changes in your sleep patterns unrelated to the typical disruptions caused by caring for a newborn during the past two weeks?

- 0: No changes

- 1: Slight changes

- 2: Moderate changes

- 3: Significant changes

Question 4

How has your appetite changed in the last two weeks?

- 0: No changes

- 1: Slight changes

- 2: Moderate changes

- 3: Significant changes

Question 5

Over the past two weeks, how often have you felt intense irritability or anger?

- 0: Not at all

- 1: Occasionally

- 2: Frequently

- 3: Most of the time

Question 6

How often have you experienced persistent fatigue or energy loss in the last two weeks?

- 0: Not at all

- 1: Occasionally

- 2: Frequently

- 3: Most of the time

Question 7

Have you had difficulty concentrating or making decisions in the last two weeks?

- 0: Not at all

- 1: Occasionally

- 2: Frequently

- 3: Most of the time

Question 8

Have you noticed any unexplained physical symptoms, such as headaches or stomachaches, in the last two weeks?

- 0: No symptoms

- 1: Slight symptoms

- 2: Moderate symptoms

- 3: Significant symptoms

Question 9

Have you withdrawn from family and friends during the past two weeks or avoided social interactions?

- 0: Not at all

- 1: Occasionally

- 2: Frequently

- 3: Most of the time

Question 10

Have you experienced intrusive, negative thoughts, particularly related to self-doubt, guilt, or thoughts of harming yourself or your baby in the last two weeks?

- 0: Not at all

- 1: Occasionaly

- 2: Frequently

- 3: Most of the time

Scoring

Add up the scores for each question to get your total score. The higher the total score, the more critical it is to discuss your feelings with a healthcare professional:

- 0–5: Low risk

- 6–10: Mild symptoms

- 11–15: Moderate symptoms

- 16–20: Significant symptoms

This self-assessment quiz is intended for informational purposes only. If you have concerns about your mental health, please consult with a healthcare professional for a thorough evaluation and appropriate guidance.

Seeking Support

It doesn't matter if you have PPD or postnatal anxiety (PNA). It can happen to any mom at any time, no matter who they are or where they come from. Women who have never had worry or sadness can be cut down at the knees soon after giving birth or even months later. It's essential to keep the conversation going about PND/PNA because "normalizing" anxiety and depression will save lives and get rid of the shame effect. It is essential to know the difference between what is expected and what is PPD, PNA, or another mental illness.

PPD

About one in seven women have PND when symptoms persist for more than two weeks and cause significant impairment in daily life. Typical signs of PND are

- a dull, sad, or low mood

- crying a lot

- losing interest in fun things

- having trouble sleeping (not because your baby is waking up)

- sleeping too much

- losing or gaining weight

- having an increased appetite

PNA

PNA is thought to happen more often than PND. A recent study found that one in five women had at least one type of worry problem while they were pregnant or after giving birth (Uduchucku, 2021). Some of the most common PNA signs are

- worry, fear, or anxiety that you can't control, like about your baby's health

- feeling irritated, tense, restless, or on edge

- having a faster heart or breathing rate than normal

- sickness or the shakes

- having trouble sleeping at night, even when your baby is asleep

- checking on your baby too much

Let me share with you my own anxiety issues during postpartum more clearly as a mom who didn't know much about PPD. I was 30 years old when I got pregnant with my child. I had a trouble-free pregnancy, but I had to have an emergency cesarean after over 30 hours of labor. My baby was born healthy, but I had trouble nursing, which caused me to worry about my milk supply and caused my infant to lose a lot of weight in the first week. I saw my physician two weeks after giving birth to get comfort regarding my C-section incision. While the incision showed no infection, the obstetrician observed a difference in my behavior. Tearful and voicing concern for my kid's well-being, I was battling with sleep and persistent thoughts of possible damage to me and my daughter.

I was sent to the OB social worker after I denied suffering from depression. I was exhausted from lack of sleep, anxious about my baby's health, and unable to leave them with anyone else. I, despite my mother's encouragement, struggled with intrusive thoughts, such as worrying that my baby might suffocate in their bed linens while I was gone. This narrative reflects the difficulties many women encounter postpartum. Several significant life events occur at once during this period, including healing after childbirth, learning to nurse, figuring out how to be a parent, and determining whether or not anything needs medical attention or is just normal. Helping new moms like myself maintain our mental health requires acknowledging and resolving such difficulties.

Being a new mother is challenging in and of itself, but imagine doing it while feeling so depressed and frightened that you no longer recognize your humanity. Just because someone you know isn't feeling 100% right after giving birth doesn't mean they won't eventually. Help her in whatever way you can, including taking her to the doctor or encouraging her to go for a walk. Suffering from anxiety or depression can be fatal, but help is available. Always grasp onto the light, and never let go of hope; your child needs you.

Where to Find Support

Are you still looking for a way to work through how you're feeling? If so, you might find it helpful to get some professional help. Still not sure if postpartum or maternal mental health therapy is right for you? Here are some things to think about:

- **Support from loved ones:** Friends and family are our main sources of emotional and practical support. Tell your loved ones how you feel and what you need. Having caring people in your life may lighten the load and foster your health and happiness.

- **Professional support:** Obstetricians, therapists, and counselors are just a few of the health workers who can help you in a way that fits your needs. Individual counseling gives you a one-on-one space to talk about and work through specific issues, while group therapy lets you connect with other moms who are going through the same things you are. Teletherapy and mental health apps are two online tools that make it easy to get professional help.

Benefits of Individual Counseling

- **Personalized care:** Individual therapy lets you have focused, one-on-one conversations about your problems and experiences.

- **Confidentiality:** This is a safe place to talk about your thoughts without fear of being judged, which builds trust and a sense of safety.

- **Goal-oriented:** Working with a therapist one-on-one lets you set and reach specific mental health and well-being goals.

Benefits of Group Therapy

- **Sharing experiences:** Talking to other moms experiencing the same problems can help you feel less alone and more like you're part of a group.

- **Validation:** Peers in group treatment who may have been through similar things can validate and understand what you're going through.

- **Diverse points of view:** Hearing different viewpoints can help you better understand coping processes and tactics.

Online Resources

In this digital age, online tools are becoming increasingly helpful in getting mental health help. Online support groups, mental health apps, and teletherapy meetings give people— especially busy moms—the freedom and flexibility they need.

Benefits of Online Resources

Being a mother today comes with problems that mothers did not have to deal with in the past. The internet and social media can provide helpful information for making decisions:

- **Accessibility:** Online tools let you get help from the comfort of your home, so you don't have to worry about things like getting somewhere or finding time to do it.

- **Flexibility:** Teletherapy allows you to schedule meetings around your schedule, making it easier to fit mental health care into your life as a new parent.

- **A level of secrecy:** Online support groups provide anonymity, which may encourage members to talk and share freely.

Remember that asking for help is a sign of strength, and you don't have to handle your complicated feelings after giving birth alone. Getting help from family, friends, and experts can make this time better and more satisfying. If you have severe signs or worries, don't wait to get help and advice from registered healthcare experts. Your health and happiness are essential; help can help you during this change.

Self-Care Practices for Emotional Well-Being

New mothers need to make time for self-care, even in the middle of the chaos of becoming a parent for the first time. Taking care of yourself has a multiplier impact on your mental health, benefiting both you and your child. Important things for self-care are set out below.

Relaxation Techniques

Relaxation methods should be part of your daily life. Deep breathing, gradual muscle relaxation, and guided images are all practices that can help you feel calm and less stressed. Spend a few minutes daily on these methods to make a quiet place for yourself.

Mindfulness Exercises

Doing awareness activities can help you stay in the present. Mindful breathing or walking can help you become more aware, lowering your stress and making you more emotionally intense. Doing things that make you aware can help you enjoy the special times of being a parent.

Journaling

Consider maintaining a notebook to write down your ideas and feelings. This reflective practice may serve as an avenue for therapeutic work, assisting you in working through the ups and downs of parenting. Record the times you are grateful, write down the times you are frustrated, and keep a log of your emotional journey. Writing in a journal can be an effective method for introspection and the catharsis of pent-up feelings.

Prioritizing Personal Needs

- Remember to put your requirements first among all the pressures of caring for your infant.

- Schedule time for self-care, such as taking a relaxing bath, reading a book, or sipping a cup of tea in peace.

- Recognize that taking care of your health directly and positively influences your capacity to care for your child.

Warning Against Burnout

Even though being a mother brings immeasurable pleasure, the obligations might sometimes seem too much. Identifying the warning symptoms of burnout and seeking assistance without delay is essential. Continuous acts of self-sacrifice without pauses might leave you exhausted and harm your overall health. Realize that taking care of yourself is not a luxury but a need to maintain a healthy lifestyle.

If you include these self-care techniques in your routine, you are laying a foundation for emotional well-being that you will pass on to your child. A well-rested and emotionally stable mother is better positioned to give the kind of love and care necessary for her child's healthy growth. Remember that your health is essential, and caring for yourself will help you develop the resilience you'll need for motherhood's incredible adventure.

Chapter 4:

Optimal Nutrition for Recovery

and Well-Being

Eating well can be challenging in this busy world, where fast food and unhealthy snacks are everywhere. Now, picture yourself as a great mom who has to work, care for a baby, and try to eat some vegetables between meetings. It's more complex! Everyone should eat well, but moms should do it even more during pregnancy and after giving birth. In their superhero mode, moms often forget to eat or grab unhealthy snacks. This could make them tired and could even be bad for their health.

Imagine a mother carrying a briefcase in one hand, a baby in the other, and a kale smoothie in a beverage container that she keeps tucked beneath her laptop. Moms who try to keep up with their careers, their children, and their social lives frequently find themselves nutritionally deficient, which may lead to health problems, weariness, and the odd "Where did I put my keys?" moments.

So, to all the superhero moms, this is your guide to eating the right, balanced food that gives you nutrition and energy. Because, let's be honest, life gets a bit crazy, and if we can't laugh about it, we might cry into a bowl of cereal. Grab a healthy snack, put on your superhero cape (real or imaginary), and let's figure out how to eat well in this wild adventure of motherhood. After all, a happy, well-fed mom is a superhero in her own right—and who knows, your baby might join in the giggles!

Postpartum Dietary Requirements

As a new mom, you may want to return to the shape you were in before you got pregnant. New moms often rush to lose the weight they gained during pregnancy. However, taking things slowly and sticking to postpartum dietary recommendations is essential for staying healthy and happy after giving birth.

Take it easy for a while after giving birth and nourish your body to help it recover. Many new mothers have trouble deciding what to eat in those first few weeks. A wide range of physical adjustments and difficulties might arise during pregnancy and childbirth.

Postpartum is a transforming time for new moms, defined by the pleasure of bringing a new life into the world alongside the bodily modifications that occur with childbirth. To effectively navigate this period, you will need to take a considered approach to eating, taking into account the additional demands placed on your body for recovery and lactation.

Let's explore postpartum nutrition further since it can affect a new mother's recovery from delivery and ability to care for her new baby. Read on to discover why postpartum nutrition is crucial and how to choose the proper meals for one's unique requirements.

Additional Calories

Immediately after giving birth, your body starts the fantastic process of healing and recovering. It is essential to provide it with the right amount of energy. Even though everyone has different calorie needs, it is usually suggested that nursing moms eat an extra 500 calories every day. With these extra calories, the body can heal and meet its energy needs while breastfeeding. Age, weight, height, and activity level influence the recommended daily calorie consumption for a healthy, moderately active woman. To clarify the recommended calorie intake, refer to the table below (Centers for Disease Control and Prevention, n.d.-c; U.S.

Department of Health and Human Services and U.S. Department of Agriculture, 2015).

Age group	Activity level	Daily calorie intake
Younger women (19–30)	Sedentary	1,800–2,000 calories
	Moderately active	2,000–2,200 calories
	Active	2,200–2,400 calories
Adult women (31–50)	Sedentary	1,800–2,000 calories
	Moderately active	2,000–2,200 calories
	Active	2,200 – 2,400 calories
Older women (51+)	Sedentary	1,600–1,800 calories
	Moderately active	1,800–2,000 calories
	Active	2,000–2,200 calories
Lactating women	Moderately active	2,300–2,500 calories

This table shows the daily recommended caloric intake women of different ages and activity levels should consume. It focuses on the extra calories breastfeeding women who do light exercise should consume.

Protein

Protein is essential for making breast milk, healing cells, and strengthening the immune system. Women who have recently given birth should try to eat more protein, approximately 25g daily (Wolf, 2019), preferably from lean sources like chicken, fish, beans, and nuts.

Eating protein-rich foods can help your muscles heal and strengthen you during this physically challenging time.

Consuming nutritious amounts of good fats, proteins, and carbs is necessary to maintain healthy milk production and nourish your body.

For instance, eggs and fatty fish are good sources of protein and healthy fats. On the other hand, vegetables, whole grains, and fruits offer sources of carbohydrates that are high in fiber. Additional healthy-fat foods include nuts, seeds, avocados, and yogurt made with full-fat milk (Lindberg, 2020).

Essential Nutrients for Recovery and Lactation

The postpartum period requires a wide variety of vital nutrients to assist in healing and satisfy the nutritional requirements of a nursing infant. Iron, zinc, and folate are three of the most critical players. Iron helps avoid anemia, zinc is essential for immunological function, and folate supports tissue regeneration (Aoki et al., 2022). A diet including various nutrient-dense foods is necessary to ensure that these requirements are satisfied.

Iron

It's possible for mothers who lose a lot of blood during labor to have trouble breathing, feel weak and tired, and even lose their appetite after giving birth. This might be because they don't have enough iron. It's also possible for your body to keep bleeding after giving birth. Iron is crucial for your body to make new blood cells by replacing the old ones.

To ensure your body can replace the iron it lost during labor, you can eat iron-rich foods after birth, like lean meat, liver, clams, oysters, enriched cereal, and green leafy veggies. If you are a vegetarian, your doctor may tell you to take iron pills.

Zinc

Zinc supplementation given after delivery greatly enhances maternal blood zinc levels and significantly reduces the chance of developing PPD (Aoki et al., 2022).

Vitamin B12 and Folate

Due to the increased nutritional requirements of the mother, the fetus, and the newborn during this time, women who are pregnant or who have just given birth, as well as women who are breastfeeding, are at an incredibly high risk for vitamin B12 and folate insufficiency or deficiency. Insufficiency in vitamin B12 and folate has significant adverse effects on public health, particularly for the health of mothers and their newborns. Anemia, abnormalities in the neurological system, and glossitis were shown to be connected with a low status of vitamin B12 and folate. Infants get their vitamin B12 and folate through breast milk. Inadequate levels of vitamin B12 in babies may result in failure to thrive, developmental regression, and severe neuropathy. Adequate levels of vitamin B12 in neonates are crucial for infants' growth and cognitive development (Shen et al., 2022).

Clams, tuna, liver, beef, and salmon are some excellent animal foods to consume to get your daily dose of vitamin B12. Vitamin B12 may also be found in some fortified cereals and dairy products. If you cannot consume meat or are a vegetarian, you may want to consider adding a B12 supplement to your diet (Reinagel, 2019).

DHA

DHA and other omega-3 fatty acids are essential because our bodies don't make enough of them by itself. DHA is an integral part of brain tissue that helps you concentrate, lowers inflammation, and reduces your risk of PPD. Even though having more DHA might not completely protect against PPD, having more DHA can help you control your emotions because it helps make serotonin. Fish like salmon and sardines, fortified eggs, and cheese are all good sources of DHA. You can get also this nutrient into your body by taking a DHA supplement.

Choline

Like folic acid, choline is an essential vitamin for brain growth. Nursing moms need to get enough of this vitamin while breastfeeding. Choline is very important for babies' brain and memory growth. The best sources are eggs, organ meats, and liver.

Vitamin D

Also known as the "sunshine vitamin," this helps the mother's body recover after childbirth by bolstering her immune, brain, and nerve systems. Fatty fish, such as egg yolks, salmon and tuna, liver, fortified dairy, and orange juice, are some of the finest dietary sources of vitamin D (Reinagel, 2019).

Postpartum nutrition is essential for all new parents, but nursing mothers must ensure their milk supply is rich in vitamins and minerals.

Superfoods for Healing and Energy

Have you ever heard the expression, "You are what you eat"? It's more like, "You need what you eat!" in the postpartum phase. Moms who are postpartum should adhere to a diet that is nutritionally sound and contains a wide variety of foods, including whole grains, vegetables, fruits, lean proteins, and healthy fats. Below, we will investigate how these food categories help your recovery and provide the essential nutrients for you and your bundle of joy. Every mom's birth story is different, and whether you had a C-section or a vaginal birth, you need help and time to heal after giving birth. For obvious reasons, you need to feed your body foods that heal and provide you with energy. Some superfoods for healing and energy are as follows.

Vitamin C

Vitamin C is one of the key essential nutrients for healthy skin. It helps make collagen and speeds up the healing of the skin's top layer. It is a potent antioxidant that also helps protect skin cells and keep your immune system in great shape. Studies have proven that vitamin C supplements can help wounds heal faster, stop keloid formation (when scars form too quickly), and boost collagen production (Grao, 2019). Adding more vitamin C to your diet can also make your skin more elastic, less wrinkled, less rough, and more even in color.

Some foods that are high in vitamin C are acerola, Kakadu plums, amla fruit, kiwifruit, papaya, bell peppers, and broccoli.

Vitamin A

Vitamin A is essential for wound healing and your baby's eyesight, overall health, and brain development. It would be best to have more vitamin A when you're nursing. When skin is damaged, vitamin A speeds up the rate at which cells fix themselves and rebuild the skin's structure Vitamin A not only helps with the inflammatory part of wound healing, but it also makes more collagen.

Goji berries and orange and yellow fruits like apples, bananas, sweet potatoes, and plums are good food sources of vitamin A. Also, dark leafy greens are a great way to get vitamins A and C.

Bromelain

This is an enzyme found in pineapple juice and skin. Evidence shows it can help ease pain, shorten recovery time after surgery, and speed up wound healing (Nall, 2023). Although bromelain is found in pineapples, the studies examining its effectiveness used a high supplement dose.

Now that you know about the nutrients, do you want to know about something that can make scars look better? Apply vitamin E or rosehip oil (high in vitamin C) to scars. These oils are also great for stretch marks (McDermott, 2023).

- Include a range of lean meats, fruits, whole grains, vegetables, and healthy fats in your diet. Sticking to complete, natural meals will ensure that you obtain the vitamins, minerals, and fiber your body needs to keep going strong while breastfeeding.

- Meat, poultry, fish, eggs, dairy, beans, nuts, and seeds are all great protein sources, and people should eat them at least twice daily.

- Consume daily fruit servings of two portions.

- It would be best to consume whole grains daily, such as those found in oatmeal, cereal, pasta, and bread.

- Fill up on leafy greens and bright yellow veggies three times a day.

- Choose salmon for its omega-3 content, which boosts brain function and reduces inflammation.

- Walnuts—like mini-brains—fuel your intellect and body. Due to their omega-3 and antioxidant content, walnuts are excellent energy foods.

Therefore, moms, adding this superfood to your meals after giving birth can help you heal by providing nutrients and energy.

Things to Avoid When Breastfeeding

Breastfeeding parents should be aware of items that might harm their babies and milk production if consumed in high amounts. Things to avoid—at least in part—when nursing are as follows.

Fish

All fish contain some mercury, a common pollutant and a known neurotoxin that can hurt a baby's brain. However, the health benefits of eating fish, including its high protein and low fat, usually outweigh the risks. If breastfeeding, you should never eat shark, swordfish, tilefish, or king mackerel, because they are the top predator fish and therefore contain the most mercury.

Alcohol

Although it's safer not to drink while nursing, it's not illegal to drink alcohol when breastfeeding. According to the American Academy of Pediatrics (AAP), you should wait about two to three hours after drinking one alcoholic drink (5 ounces of wine, one shot of alcohol, or 12 ounces of beer) before breastfeeding or pumping (*Pump and Dump: Is It Necessary After Drinking?*, n.d.). This is so your body has time to break down the alcohol. If you don't, the alcohol could get into your baby's system through your breast milk.

Caffeine

These days, most moms are hooked on coffee, which is a stimulant that can get into breast milk and affect a baby's growth or make them jittery. It's in tea, coffee, chocolate, a lot of soft drinks, and over-the-counter drugs. It's good to consume caffeine in moderation while nursing. You should not have more than three cups of coffee, soft drinks, or tea daily. Instead of coffee, drink about 96 ounces of water daily, which is about 10 to 12 eight-ounce cups (*Postpartum Nutrition: What to Eat After You Give Birth?*, 2022).

Meal Planning and Preparation Tips

During the chaos of making changes after giving birth, meal planning becomes like a superhero power, especially for moms doing many things at once, like working and being a mom. Planning meals for the week guarantees a varied and healthy menu and presents the idea of cooking in large batches, which is the most convenient way to cook. This is a massive help for moms who work outside the home. Imagine having a week's worth of meals planned and ready to go, just waiting to be warmed up. It's a beauty that saves time, reduces stress, and improves nutrition. The key is planning, giving yourself time each week to make a food plan, cooking a batch, and enjoying having tasty choices ready. This method not only meets the food needs of new moms but also makes the time after giving birth more accessible and fun. So start making plans for mealtimes so they are well-thought-out and stress-free:

- Use batch cooking brilliance to make prepping a significant amount of food more accessible. In this way, busy people can spend more time on other duties throughout the week while still eating well. Batch cooking reduces stress, boosts energy, and improves health.

- Use freezer-friendly cooking, often known as the art of freezing meals, to have a supply of nutritious options.

- You can save valuable preparation time by cutting and washing vegetables before use. Make sure that you have an adequate supply of these time-saving components so that you can quickly prepare nutritious meals.

- Involve any friends or family members who are available to help prepare meals.

As a new parent, one of your primary responsibilities is caring for your body and your infant. So this is it: The dietary example below is designed with your health in mind. It includes seven days' worth of healthful, filling, and simple-to-prepare meals.

Sample Meal Plan

Day	Breakfast	Lunch	Dinner
1	Overnight oats with Greek yogurt, berries, and chia seeds	Quinoa salad with chickpeas, veggies, and feta cheese	Slow cooker chicken stew with mixed vegetables and brown rice
2	Whole-grain toast with avocado and poached egg	Lentil soup with spinach and tomatoes	Baked salmon with roasted sweet potatoes and asparagus

3	Greek yogurt smoothie with spinach, banana, and almond butter	Quinoa and black bean bowl with avocado	Vegetable stir-fry with tofu and brown rice
4	Chia pudding with mango and coconut milk	Turkey and veggie wrap with whole-grain tortilla	Baked ziti with whole-wheat pasta and tomato sauce
5	Vegetable omelets with spinach and tomatoes	Quinoa bowl with roasted vegetables and feta cheese	Slow cooker chickpea curry with basmati rice
6	Whole-grain pancakes with fresh berries	Chicken and vegetable stir-fry with brown rice	Grilled shrimp salad with quinoa and avocado
7	Avocado toast with poached egg	Spinach and feta stuffed bell peppers	Vegetable lasagna with whole-wheat noodles

This example meal plan is a tool that will make postpartum nutrition easier, enabling you to concentrate on what matters most—caring for yourself and your darling infant—instead of having to figure out what to eat. Suppose a nursing woman follows a diet plan designed for lactating mothers. In that case, it may help ensure she is getting the appropriate amount of calories, protein, vitamins, and minerals for her personal well-being and her child's development.

Supplements

The time after delivery is a transitional phase that requires a heightened focus on diet to facilitate the most successful recovery. Although eating a well-rounded diet should be the starting point, nutritional supplements may also be essential to ensure new moms get the necessary nutrients. This section will address the function of several supplements, namely calcium, vitamin D, and iron, in facilitating postpartum recovery.

Calcium Supplements

Calcium is essential for maintaining bone health, particularly during the postpartum recovery period. To reinforce your diet and support healing and breastfeeding, you should investigate the many supplement alternatives available, such as calcium carbonate and citrate.

Vitamin D Supplements

Vitamin D, sometimes known as the "sunshine vitamin," is integral in several biological activities, making it a critical component of postpartum health. It can be obtained via sunlight. Understanding the necessity of vitamin D supplementation becomes more urgent as new moms juggle the demands of recovery and nursing because it influences bone health, immunity, and potential mental well-being.

Iron Supplements

Iron is an essential mineral, particularly after childbirth when the body is going through a period of tremendous transition. Understanding the significance of iron supplements may be of great assistance when it comes to maintaining energy and fostering a good recovery for new moms. Hemoglobin is the molecule in the blood that carries oxygen, and iron is a crucial part of it. Two of the most prevalent difficulties in the postpartum period are low hemoglobin levels and exhaustion. Postpartum tiredness can be reduced, and physical endurance improved, with the help of iron supplements. Iron helps the body use oxygen more efficiently, which boosts energy and speeds up the healing process.

New moms can navigate a solid and fulfilling postpartum experience with the help of well-chosen supplements. As the healing process progresses, the nutritional assistance from these supplements will be a shining example of your dedication to your overall health, guaranteeing that the radiance of new motherhood will shine brightly for years to come.

Chapter 5:

Breastfeeding 101—From

Challenges to Success

As modern moms, we're well-prepared with the classes that teach us about labor, the postpartum period, and even the best positions for breastfeeding. Yet, when it comes to applying those positions in real-life scenarios, it can be a struggle. But let's talk about the great things about breastfeeding: It's a natural way for you and your baby to bond and has many benefits including less bleeding after giving birth, a lower chance of breast and ovarian cancer, and a faster return to the weight you were before you got pregnant. Remember that, even though we're busy, we are also on-the-go meals for our little ones—like a restaurant that's open 24/7. Your cute customer (your baby!) always insists on the chef's specialty: the magical breast milk stew. So, dear moms of today, consider this your go-to solution for feeding challenges. And for those just starting this journey, let's discuss any hiccups that might come your way during this phase. You've got this!

The ability to nourish and support your baby with what your body produces is nothing short of miraculous, and the snug bonding time provides you and your little one with all of the lovely sensations (literally). Breastfeeding is an incredible thing. Keeping this in mind, we are all aware that nursing isn't always a glamorous experience, and there are instances when it isn't even all that enjoyable!

Common Breastfeeding Challenges and Solutions

Breastfeeding is more accessible for some women than it is for others, but it's never a walk in the park. It may be tricky (and, yes, even painful) for some moms who are trying to breastfeed their children. Some first-time mothers may even berate themselves, convinced it is their fault that they cannot figure out something that seems to come so quickly to most other mothers. Before you give up and decide to quit nursing, it is essential to keep in mind that, just as with everything new at the beginning, there is a learning curve involved with breastfeeding.

When mothers leave the hospital, one of the most significant factors that contributes to their difficulty in nursing is that they do not have enough access to breastfeeding information and support during the critical first week. The lack of complete information about these issues makes it more likely that big problems will appear.

Every mother has her obstacles when she first starts nursing her child. In this section, we'll discuss some of the most frequent problems mothers have during nursing and provide you with actionable advice for overcoming them.

Low Milk Supply

Many women worry that they aren't making enough breast milk or that their milk isn't coming in. However, most of the time, your body makes just what your baby needs. It would be best if you massaged your breasts a lot in the first few hours, days, and weeks to help them start making milk. Not having enough breast milk is pretty uncommon. Other factors, such as not nursing often enough, adding formula without first pumping your breasts, having an inadequate latch, taking certain drugs, your baby being born early, or having high blood pressure during pregnancy, might more often than not create issues with milk production or breastfeeding.

- **Ideally, breastfeeding should occur every three hours:** During the first two weeks of life, your infant will eat 8–12 times per 24 hours. Do not miss feedings or pumping sessions; instead, pay attention to your infant's indications and allow them to inform you when it is time to eat.

- **When feeding or pumping, use your hands:** Hand expression is one of the most effective strategies to boost milk supply in nursing mothers.

- **Always offer both breasts during nursing:** It is perfectly normal for your child to consume milk from just one breast at times, but if this behavior becomes routine, it will cause your breast milk supply to drop. Pumping the second breast may help ease pressure on your breasts and safeguard your milk supply while you wait for your baby to eat more at each meal.

- **When your baby is young, bottles and pacifiers should be avoided:** If you start giving your child bottles or pacifiers too soon, your child may have nipple confusion. Babies may have difficulty transitioning between nursing and eating from a bottle, which can interfere with their capacity to latch onto the breast correctly.

- **Certain drugs need a discussion with your doctor:** Certain approaches to hormonal contraception, including birth control pills and antihistamines like Benadryl and Zyrtec, may significantly reduce a nursing mother's ability to produce milk.

- **Focus on yourself:** Get as much rest as possible, eat healthily, abstain from alcohol and nicotine, maintain a healthy hydration level, and allow people to assist you.

Engorgement (Stiff, Sore, and Painful Breast Swelling)

Some new moms worry they won't make enough milk, while others feel like they are about to burst. When your breasts are full of milk, they usually get bigger, heavier, and slightly sore. This usually occurs in the early days when your milk starts to come in and is not removed efficiently. The breasts will become overfull, partly with milk, partly with increased tissue fluid and blood, which interfere with milk flow. The mother may have a fever, with rock-hard swollen breasts, making it challenging for the baby to latch on. This usual fullness in your breasts will go away over the next few days as your body gets used to supplying your baby's needs. Engorgement can cause a clogged duct or a breast infection, so it's best to try to avoid it before it happens.

Tips to Relieve your Symptoms

- Before each feeding, apply a warm, wet compress to your breasts and massage them for two to three minutes.

- Ice may be used up to 20 minutes after feedings to reduce swelling and discomfort.

- Nipples shouldn't be treated with moist heat or ice.

Mastitis and Fungal Infections

Breast infections, or mastitis, are often caused by germs entering via a broken nipple. Suddenly, you may feel a hardening, reddening, warming, or soreness in your breasts. Late symptoms include red streaks, fever, and flu-like symptoms.

You should contact a doctor and start taking an oral antibiotic, but it's okay to continue breastfeeding. In most cases, breastfeeding effectively eliminates the infection and unblocks the duct.

Another typical issue for nursing mothers is thrush, a fungal infection. An overabundance of yeast is to blame for this illness. White patches may appear inside your baby's cheeks, tongue, and gums, making your nipples and breasts hurt.

If you suspect thrush, it's best to contact both your doctor and the doctor your baby sees so you can get a proper diagnosis and treatment for both of you at the same time. This will reduce the likelihood of spreading the disease further.

Sore Nipples

As you and your baby become used to nursing, you may experience sensitivity or tenderness in your nipples. Breastfeeding shouldn't be painful, despite what you may have heard. Once you and your baby have settled into a few excellent nursing positions and the latch is secure, breastfeeding should be rather pleasant.

Tips to Reduce Nipple Pain

- Ensure that the latch is working properly. If your baby is correctly latched, your nipple and at least half of your areola should be sucked into your baby's mouth. This will let you know that your baby is adequately latched. If the latch is not closed completely, you will probably feel a pinch (ouch!), and you might end up with painful or cracked nipples as a result. If, after one minute of breastfeeding, you are still experiencing discomfort, gently push a clean finger into the corner of your baby's mouth to break the seal. Then, try nursing your baby again, ensuring their mouth is wide open.

- To put pressure on a different part of the breast, try moving around while you nurse.

- If your clothes and bras are too tight, they will put pressure on your nipples.

- Do not put solid soaps or creams on your nipples. Before bed, let your nipples air dry and express a little breast milk. This will help them heal and stay healthy.

- Talk to your doctor or a breastfeeding expert if the pain doesn't go away.

Inverted, Flat, or Huge Nipples

Women's nipples come in many shapes and sizes, just like belly buttons. If your nipples are flat, turn inward, or are very big, it can be hard to nurse, but there are ways to fix this. No matter what shape or size your nipple is, most babies can still latch on and nurse. If you're scared that your baby isn't latching on well because of your nipple, talk to your healthcare provider or a lactation expert. They can help you and your baby get used to things.

Tongue-Tie

Your baby's healthcare practitioner or a qualified lactation consultant are the only people who can identify your baby as having tongue-tie. However, tongue-tie may lead to issues with latching, painful nipples, and irritability in your baby. When a newborn has a tongue-tie, it means that the tissue connecting the floor of their mouth to the front of their tongue is either too short or stretches too far forward.

Baby Gassy or Fussy After Feeding

If your baby is unhappy, incredibly fussy, or gassy after feedings, they may be gulping or swallowing a lot of air, suggesting they are not correctly latched. During breastfeeding or bottle feeding, all newborns will swallow some air, but the best method to assist them with gas is to ensure your baby has a good latch to prevent them from consuming too much air. Here are some more things that can help:

- Make sure to give your child a good burp when changing breasts and at the end of each feeding.

- Refrain from overfeeding your baby or feeding them too rapidly.

- Think about the foods you eat. Many moms are afraid that the foods they eat make their children gassy.

Dealing with these problems with patience and the right tools can make nursing an excellent and satisfying experience. Each woman's breastfeeding journey is unique, so you may or may not have any of these issues (Olsson, 2022).

Latching and Positioning Techniques

Breastfeeding is a beautiful way to nourish your child. A healthy, full-term infant will likely learn how to breastfeed automatically. While breastfeeding may come quickly to some mothers, others achieve mastery of it more slowly. If your baby can't latch on properly, it can be frustrating, make you feel guilty, and cause stress. Even though breastfeeding seems like it should be the easiest thing in the world, it may take some trial and error before you and your baby discover the ideal position for nursing success.

Each mother learns what works best for her and her child, and these methods may vary. Learning to latch and place your baby for optimal feeding is like mastering complex ballet steps. Picture it as a ballet, with your small one as your darling dancing partner. Let's have fun while learning the nuances of appropriate latching and placing with this spin.

Positioning

Like learning new dancing movements, there is beauty in trying out various nursing positions. Breastfeeding can be done in one of four standard positions. Newborns are often easier to handle in the football and cross-cradle grips, while mothers who have recently had a cesarean section may find the side-lying position more to their liking. An older infant who is good at latching and can support their head in the cradle hold may find this position more comfortable position. Try out several options to discover the one that works best for you.

Before picking a position, make sure you are as relaxed as possible. For example, go to the bathroom before you start, because you may be feeding for a long time! If you want to nurse, find something to support your back and have a pillow close by to position your baby at breast level. Keep a glass of water close by because breastfeeding moms get thirsty.

Football Hold/Rugby Position

In this position, your baby's head is on your breast, and their body is tucked under your arm, next to your back. If you had a cesarean birth, this position is recommended after giving birth since it keeps your baby away from the incision. The majority of babies feel very at ease when held in this manner. If you have a strong milk ejection reflex (letdown), this position is also beneficial since your infant will have an easier time managing the milk flow.

Cradle Hold

- If you want to breastfeed your child while rocking them in a cradle or holding them across your lap, your child should be positioned so they are lying on their side, with their shoulder and hip supported, and their mouth should be at the same level as your nipple. The whole of their front body must contact your front body.

- Particularly in the first few weeks after your baby's birth, you should use cushions to elevate your infant and support your elbows to get your baby up to breast height.

- Use the "U" grip or the "C" hold to support your breast. Your baby's head will rest on your forearm, and their back will run down the inside of your arm and the palm of your hand. You ought to be able to see your baby's back when you look down.

- Your baby's lips should hide a half-inch or more of the shadowy region surrounding your breast. Check that your baby's ear, shoulder, and hips are aligned in the same direction. As a newborn, the top and bottom of your baby's head should be at the same level.

Cross-Cradle

- To breastfeed your child while seated in this position, you must place a cushion across your lap and prop your child up on it so they are at the same level as your nipple. Pillows should also support both elbows so that arms are not required to maintain your baby's weight while breastfeeding; otherwise, your arms will tire before the feeding is complete.

- When you are getting ready to breastfeed on your left breast, you should support that breast with your left hand in a "U" hold position. The fingers on your right hand should be used to provide support for your infant. Switch hands if you are nursing on the other side.

- Place your hand softly behind your baby's ears and neck, then put your thumb and index finger behind their ears. Do this while your baby is awake. The web that forms between your thumb, index finger, and the palm of your hand serves as a "second neck" for your baby, and their neck should rest there. Your baby's shoulder blades should be cradled in the palm of your hand when you do this.

- When you are getting ready to latch your baby onto you, make sure that, from the very beginning, their mouth is extremely near to your nipple.

- When your baby's mouth is wide open, apply pressure between their shoulder blades using the palm of your hand. Their lips should be at least a half-inch away from the base of your nipple when they latch on to you.

Side-Lying

- After the first few days of nursing, some women find this position the most comfortable. However, it's possible that learning the other positions initially is less complicated. Working on perfecting this posture throughout the day is beneficial.

- You may also discover that lying down is the most comfortable posture when feeding during the night. You and your baby should both roll onto your sides so that you are facing each other. To make yourself more comfortable, you can position a cushion behind your back and another either behind or between your legs. You can prevent your infant from rolling away from you by placing a cushion or a rolled-up blanket behind their back. Your forearm should be positioned so your baby's back is against it while you hold them in your arm. When your infant's hips are flexed, and their ear, shoulder, and hip are aligned, it is easier for them to take in milk (*Positioning*, n.d.).

Step-by-Step Guide to Achieving a Good Latch

Starting nursing as soon as possible, preferably within 30 minutes of giving birth, will help ensure your baby latches on correctly. Skin-to-skin touch should begin immediately after birth and last for at least two hours, unless a doctor says otherwise. Skin-to-skin touch should then happen as often as possible for the first few weeks after giving birth. A partner or support person can also do skin-to-skin touch if the mother is absent.

Let's talk about the actual art now: the perfect latch which ensures the milk moves smoothly and avoids awkward slip-ups. Follow these steps:

- **Baby's mouth wide open:** Touching your baby's top lip gently with your breast can encourage a wide-open mouth position.

- **Aim for more than just the nipple:** You should make sure your infant receives a large mouthful of your breast, which should include both the nipple and a sizeable amount of the areola.

- **Listen for swallowing sounds:** Listen carefully for the lilting tune that signifies your child is getting enough nourishment from the breast milk you provide. Your infant is leading the dance and providing the beat.

- **Comfort is vital:** Examine your level of comfort. If you are experiencing any discomfort, you should try again after carefully breaking the latch. The nursing waltz is about finding the position that gives you the maximum comfort and coziness.

- **Feed on demand:** Find out when your baby is hungry by paying attention to their signs. Most of the time, these signs show up when your baby is in a quiet but alert stage. The signs are

  - during light sleep, your baby's eyes move quickly

  - moving hands and feet

  - moving hand to mouth

  - rooting (moving their head with their mouth open)

  - sucking sounds and movements

- **Always remember**

  - tummy to mummy

  - face to breast

  - nose to nipple

  - bottom tucked in

Remember that your nursing ballet is a one-of-a-kind performance, and no standard routine applies to everyone (*Latch and Position*, n.d.).

Breast Care and Pumping Advice

Breast stimulation and milk extraction from the breasts are the two most crucial things to do to maintain a healthy supply of milk. When it is not feasible for a person to breastfeed their child, they can use a breast pump device to express (extract) milk from their breasts. Many mothers use a breast pump to pump their breast milk so they can continue to supply their infant with breast milk even when they are separated from their child, such as when they have to return to work or school or when their child is sick. Whether you breastfeed your child or use a pump, breast milk offers several advantages for your baby.

Moms need to maintain good care for their breasts while feeding their babies through pumping. Follow the steps below:

- Before you pump, wash your hands with soap and water for at least 20 seconds.

- Breast hygiene is also crucial because an unclean breast contains germs and bacteria. Always wash the nipple area with clean water before breastfeeding.

- Clean the pump's buttons and any areas close by.

- Ensure the parts of the pump and the containers for collecting milk are clean. It's not necessary to sterilize the pump or bottles when pumping for a healthy baby; wash them with hot, warm water. Do not let the parts of the pump soak in water between uses. Instead, rinse them and let them dry.

- A lot of people like to sit down while they pump. For electric pumps, make sure the pressure is just right. It shouldn't hurt to pump. Some pumps let you change the spinning speed, which is the number of pumping cycles per minute. Some people initially set the speed to be fast, then slowly lower it as their milk starts to flow steadily.

Some people have trouble with letdown when they're pumping. This means that they can only see drops of milk coming out of their nipples instead of streams of milk. If this happens to you, you should take good care of your breasts and try these things to help them let down:

- Before you pump, rub your breasts gently.

- Before you pump, put a clean, warm, wet cloth over your breasts.

- Pump in a dark, quiet place to avoid being interrupted.

- Look at a picture of your child or smell their blanket.

- Water or a warming pack wrapped around the breast pump's handle will warm it.

Storing Breast Milk

The temperature at which breast milk is kept depends on several factors, including whether or not the infant is healthy and whether or not you want to offer the milk to your baby immediately. Breast milk can be safely kept in the following manner for infants who are well and being cared for at home:

- At room temperature (around 77–79 °F or 25–27 °C) for up to four hours.

- If required, for up to 24 hours inside an insulated cooler with ice packs.

- In the refrigerator for a maximum of eight days (however, it has been proved that storage for up to 10 days is acceptable if the milk was pumped under extremely clean circumstances). The ideal time to keep it is between three and five days.

- You can keep it in the freezer for up to a year. Breast milk that has been thawed can be kept in a regular refrigerator for up to 24 hours without risk of spoilage. It is not recommended to refreeze milk that has previously been frozen and then thawed.

The standard for storing milk for hospitalized infants is 96 hours, equivalent to four days.

Like breastfeeding, feeding breastmilk using a bottle should take at least 10–15 minutes. The remaining milk in the bottle can be saved for another feeding for up to two hours (Enger & Hurst, 2023).

Feeding Alternatives

Every mother only wants the best for her child, but the right decisions are sometimes obscure. The old saying "breast is best" rings a bell, right? However, some mothers and infants may find it challenging to breastfeed successfully.

Not a problem. Breastfeeding isn't the only option; several others are just as healthy and safe.

Babies who are breastfed have a lower chance of needing medical care and are less likely to have problems with growth, appearance, and sleepiness.

Some mothers find it easier to decide what to put in the baby's bottle than whether to bottle feed at all. Pumped breast milk or commercial formula. Vegan or lactose-intolerant? Should I buy American or European? These thoughts will be there in all moms' heads.

Even if you're not nursing, you can still give your infant breast milk. The best kind is your own, expressed with an electronic or manual pump and refrigerated or frozen for later use. However, there are other methods available nowadays, and the labels on infant formula sold in stores will often boast about the specific ingredients and health benefits they provide.

When nursing is not an option, babies can get the nutrition they need from formula. Different formulas are designed to meet various requirements. The kind of protein and whether or not it may upset your baby's stomach are the primary factors that differentiate the different formulas:

- **Cow's-milk protein:** Protein extracted from cow's milk. Most infant formula is made from cow's milk, altered to match human breast milk.

- **Soy-based formula:** Formula made from soy is a safe and healthy alternative to dairy-based formula if your infant cannot digest dairy-based formula.

- **Hydrolyzed formulas:** These formulas have had the protein in them hydrolyzed, which means it has been broken up into tiny pieces and is thus more straightforward to digest. Formulas that have been partially hydrolyzed may alleviate some intestinal pain symptoms. If you have reason to believe that your infant suffers from food allergies, one option to consider is a formula that has been extensively hydrolyzed (Cristol, n.d.).

Formula feeding gives parents more options and ensures babies get all the nutrients they need to grow and develop. It's an option for families who are having trouble breastfeeding or who want to try something different.

Combi Feeding: Combining Breastfeeding and Formula Feeding

Combining formula feeding and breastfeeding is called "combi feeding" or "mixed feeding." For women who may be having trouble but still want to breastfeed, this method gives them options.

Benefits of Combi Feeding

- It lets moms choose between nursing and formula, which makes the feeding schedule more flexible.

- It also enables partners and other caregivers to participate in feeding, fostering a supportive environment.

Tips for Combi Feeding

- Moms can tailor a feeding plan that works for them by choosing to breastfeed at some times and using formula at other times.

- Breastfeeding mothers can keep their milk production up and supplement with formula if they want to pump and express.

Considerations

- Combi feeding is a helpful and stress-free option for women who are experiencing mental health issues.

- Combi feeding may also help mothers who need to take drugs that interfere with breastfeeding get the care they need.

Combi feeding is an intermediate option between exclusive nursing and exclusive formula feeding. It's an individualized option that promotes a positive feeding connection and the health of both mom and baby.

Deconstructing the "Breast Is Best" Myth

It's time to debunk the idea that breast milk is the sole healthy option for infants. We recognize the diversity of motherhood and celebrate the many ways in which babies can be fed and cared for.

Addressing Individual Needs

Understanding that maternal mental health and medical needs play essential roles, this chapter argues for tailored decisions that promote the well-being of both mom and baby. By being open to alternative feeding methods, we recognize the variety of ways in which parents raise their children and advocate for options that promote a prosperous and healthy start for every beautiful little one.

As a new mom, I faced the common challenge of latching difficulties during the early postnatal days. It was a struggle that left me feeling both frustrated and exhausted. My baby and I couldn't quite figure it out, and despite numerous attempts, breastfeeding didn't come as naturally as I had hoped. In those initial weeks, I had to use formula to ensure my little one got the nourishment needed. It was a tough call, but also led me to seek the proper guidance. Through conversations with a few experienced girlfriends and recommendations from supportive nurses, I gathered invaluable insights and tips. Armed with this newfound knowledge, I persevered and, gradually, my baby and I found our rhythm. The latching struggle became a triumph, a testament to the power of shared experiences and the support of those who've walked the same path. Today, our breastfeeding journey is a beautiful connection that started with challenges but blossomed into a bond strengthened by resilience and the wisdom of others.

Chapter 6:

Newborn Care Essentials

As a new mom, you have a lot of things to do. When you're getting ready for your baby to arrive, shopping for baby basics is at the top of your list. You'll need all of your stuff as soon as the baby comes. After setting up the nursery and ensuring you have everything you need for sleeping, eating, and changing diapers, it's easy to spend a lot of time getting everything that every baby needs.

Everybody adjusts to life with a newborn, and so will you. Imagine that you have organized the arrival of your little one in the same way that a superhero would prepare a surprise entry. The baby's room? Pay attention there. Baby wipes? Verify everything. But what do you think? Life following the birth of a child is similar to walking into a comedy performance in which you star as the main attraction. Suddenly, sleep becomes a rare unicorn—you hear about it, but achieving it feels like going on a magical journey. Your once quiet home turns into a 24/7 party zone hosted by your tiny new boss, who thinks sleep is optional. Now, your little CEO decides when the company meetings (aka diaper changes) happen. Forget about your old timetable, since your baby is now in charge. However, despite all the chaos of a new baby, one crucial lesson emerges: the significance of infant care essentials.

A baby needs to have a lot of things, which might surprise any parent-to-be. Want to know how to tell the difference between what you don't need for your baby and what you do? Don't worry! Let take a look below.

Newborn Hygiene and Diapering

Your baby's health and well-being depend on careful and constant care, especially regarding cleanliness. Newborn babies are very fragile and cleanliness is integral to their health. Every mom needs to know how important it is to keep things clean to ensure their baby stays healthy and happy. When providing proper care for your infant, the following details must always be kept in mind.

Bathing Your Newborn

As a new mother, bath time is more than just cleansing—it's a bonding ritual. It's essential to be gentle when bathing your baby. For your baby's comfort and health, use lukewarm water and light, fragrance-free baby soap when bath time comes around. The skin of newborns is very soft and delicate, and the sharp chemicals and strong scents in some soaps can easily hurt it.

Choosing a light baby soap with no scent lowers your baby's risk of skin irritations and allergies and keeps their skin soft and healthy. Babies should take baths in the proper water—not too hot or cold. Always stick your elbow or wrist in the water to ensure it's the right temperature for your child.

Umbilical Cord Care

When it comes to your baby's fragile umbilical cord stump, treat it with care. Avoid using harsh chemicals while cleaning it; use water and let it air dry. Until the cord stump dries and comes off, which usually takes between 10 days and three weeks, clean the surrounding area with plain water and wipe it dry. It would help to not bathe the belly button in water until the stump comes off and the region heals. It is typical for the cord stump to darken from yellow to brown or black before it comes off. If the area is red, smells terrible, or drains pus, you should see a doctor immediately (*A Guide for First-Time Parents*, n.d.).

Proper Diaper Care

Understanding the diapering dos and don'ts is essential for your baby's health and happiness. Here's a quick reference guide to assist you with this crucial part of caring for a baby:

Dos

- Always change your baby's diaper after they eat or poop, and do so regularly. Diaper rash can be avoided by always making sure your infant is dry.

- Pick diapers that are the right size and weight for your child. Diapers that don't fit properly might cause leaks and discomfort.

- Apply a light diaper cream to build a protective barrier against moisture and avoid diaper rash. Choose products that only use natural materials and have no artificial scents.

Don'ts

- Never wait until a diaper is full before changing it; this is especially important for babies. Prolonged contact with wetness might lead to skin irritation and diaper rash.

- Do not secure diapers too firmly. Ensure they fit snugly but not too tightly to provide enough ventilation and comfort.

- Check diapers regularly. Babies may have fewer obvious wettings, but they still need their diapers changed often.

Cutting Your Baby's Nails

It's essential to be careful when trimming your baby's nails so you don't accidentally hurt them. Use safe scissors for babies, wait until they are calm, and gently hold their hands. Don't cut too close to the skin to avoid cutting or nicking them by mistake. For your baby's happiness and safety, do this one easy thing: Buy nail tools or files for babies that are safe for their soft nails. These tools are smaller and have smooth edges, making it less likely that you will cut either them or yourself. Pick a time when your baby is calm, comfy, and not likely to move quickly. It's usually best to do it after a bath or while they're sleeping.

Oral Hygiene

Caring for a newborn's oral hygiene is vital even before their teeth come in. A simple way that works well is to clean their gums gently. Wipe your baby's gums with a clean, wet cloth or cotton pad after each feeding. Always be gentle because your baby's mouth is very soft and needs to be touched gently. By teaching your child these early oral hygiene habits, you're setting them up for a lifetime of good dental health.

Handling Visitors

Having friends when you have a new baby means finding the right mix between sharing your happiness and ensuring your baby is safe. An important thing to do is to ensure everyone washes their hands properly before holding your baby. In the first few months, when your baby's immune system is still growing, this simple step makes it much less likely that you will spread germs. By being careful with guests, you can ensure your baby is in a safe and calm place, giving you peace of mind during this particular time (Soni, 2023).

Figuring out how to clean and change a child is like finding the key to a happy, healthy baby.

Sleeping and Soothing Techniques

One of the most critical tasks for new parents is to help their infants develop appropriate sleep routines. Congratulations! Welcoming a new baby into the world means that you and your baby are getting used to sleeping. At this point, it might be hard to tell if either of you is having trouble sleeping because you will both be getting used to your own sleep habits and rhythms. As a new mom, you should try to sleep when your baby sleeps during the day and at night for the first few months so you can give them lots of naps and cuddles. Some children don't know how to sleep on their own. A lot of parents want to rock their babies to sleep before bed. Newborns will fall asleep while being fed.

Newborn babies usually sleep for a total of eight to nine hours during the day and eight hours at night. They have to wake up every few hours to eat because their stomachs aren't huge. Most babies don't sleep through the night (a six- to eight-hour stretch) until they are at least three months old, but this is only sometimes the case. Some babies only sleep through the night when they are almost a year old. Your newborn baby will likely be hungry and ready to eat at least once every three hours.

Between three and six months, your baby will start going to bed, napping, and waking up regularly daily. You'll learn to recognize when your baby is naturally tired and work on putting them down. If you want to do baby sleep training (sleep teaching or self-soothing training), wait until your baby is at least four to six months old. Your baby's doctor will tell you when they are physically and mentally ready.

When it comes to nap time, no two babies are the same. Children sleep at different times and for varying amounts each night and during the daytime. You may have a naturally early riser who loves to get up before the sun and feed straight away, or your kid may sleep a little longer (lucky you!).

Lullabies help to establish safe spaces for infants to get a good sleep, transforming stressful situations into calm ones. Babies may have difficulty adjusting to their new sleeping arrangements, especially if they are very different from the environment in which they were born. New parents generally have little recollection of their own infancy, making it difficult to understand their newborn's sleep patterns and preferences. As a result, I hope the following techniques will help your newborn adjust to their new world. Since your newborn has just spent nine months in the cozy confines of your womb, they are unable to understand when it's daytime or nighttime for the first few weeks of their life.

Establishing Healthy Sleep Patterns

Children who get enough restorative sleep are more likely to be happy, which makes parents happy too. The sleep cycles of infants are much shorter in duration compared to those of adults. Mothers should establish routines that promote the development of healthy sleep patterns in their newborn infants.

Creating a Soothing Sleep Environment

The sleep environment matters—a lot. When putting a baby to sleep, it's preferable to recreate the soft conditions they experienced in the womb. Swaddling, shushing, swinging, sucking, and holding your baby in the side/stomach position are the 5 S's that will help your baby sleep better. To put your child to sleep peacefully and quietly. The perfect sleeping environment includes everything from low lighting to soft blankets.

Soothing Techniques for a Fussy Baby

Fussy times are unavoidable, but fret not! Babies benefit from a relaxing sleep ritual that may include feeding, cuddling, bathing, reading, massaging, and lullabying. Don't put your infant to bed hungry. Feeding your baby every 1.5 to 2 hours throughout the day during the first few months can help them feel full and sleep through the night. Between 10 pm and midnight, provide a dream feed to aid sleep and reduce nighttime awakenings (Karp, n.d.).

Find out what helps your baby relax, whether it's the warm embrace of swaddling or the soothing sound of white noise.

Swaddling

Swaddling is a technique used to comfort and soothe babies by recreating the closeness and warmth of the womb. As a result, you'll have less trouble falling asleep and staying asleep.

- **Disadvantage:** Some infants may struggle to remain contained inside the swaddle, and it is critical to ensure that the method is performed correctly to prevent hip dysplasia.

White Noise and Pacifiers

You can create a soothing atmosphere for your child with the help of white noise, which generates a constant background sound that can cover other noises. It will mask the noises of your home and let your young one go to sleep more easily. Alternatively, pacifiers provide a nonnutritive kind of sucking comfort that, when used appropriately, may help calm a fussy infant.

- **Disadvantage:** There is a possibility that prolonged exposure to intense white noise might have an impact on your baby's hearing. It is essential to maintain the volume at an appropriate level. The excessive use of pacifiers may disrupt the nursing relationship, and some infants may develop a dependency that will be difficult to overcome in the future.

Gentle Rocking

Rocking is a method that can be used to relax an infant and put them to sleep since it mimics the motion that they experienced in the womb. It helps to create a feeling of connection as well as safety.

- **Disadvantage:** Some infants develop a need to be rocked to sleep, and abruptly stopping this routine might cause them to exhibit reluctance to fall asleep.

Let me tell you about my own journey to finding the secret of lulling my baby to a peaceful sleep. In the beginning, my evenings were filled with the familiar sound of cranky crying and the occasional period of restlessness. My husband and I were having trouble falling asleep, so I made it a point to establish a regular nighttime ritual. The three foundations of our evening routine were a soothing bath, a soft lullaby, and the warm hug of swaddling. In the end, swaddling was the saving grace of our sleep story. The tight covering provided my baby with a feeling of security akin to that experienced in the womb. Every time I said, "It's time to rest, little one" to my baby, and each warm embrace, eased them from the day's stress into the calm of slumber. This individualized combination of swaddling became a soothing experience as the weeks went into months. The infant who used to keep me up at night is now the source of gentle lullabies. My child has always slept better because of our consistent pattern, and it has become a particular time for us to connect. This sleep miracle taught me the value of patience and the skill of tailoring methods to my child's specific requirements, as every baby is different, and what works for one may not work for another.

Recognizing and Addressing Common Issues

The first few days spent with a new baby are filled with happiness, but they may also present obstacles that force parents to look for answers. Among them is the worry that your newborn may get an illness. How will you find out? It is not always easy to determine whether or not a baby is feeling well. You may need to become more familiar with your baby's typical activity patterns. Because of this, it may be challenging to determine whether or not your baby's behavior is abnormal. In neonates, the symptoms of severe illnesses can often be difficult to see, and it can be complicated to identify them.

It is essential to understand the indicators that might suggest that your infant is ill. After birth, a baby's immune system is significantly weakened, making it more difficult to ward against illnesses. When they catch an infection, their condition might rapidly deteriorate. Because of this, you need to know what to look for.

In the following sections, we will look into some of the typical problems babies may face, giving insights on spotting signs and symptoms and providing valuable tips for managing and relieving pain.

Colic

Colic is a condition characterized by an excessive amount of crying in an otherwise healthy and well-fed infant. Infants who suffer from colic often cry out uncontrollably for more than three hours on more than three days of the week.

When infants feel the urge to defecate, they may become restless, stay awake, and act as if they are in discomfort. Sometimes, they seem to have a bloated stomach, and when this happens, they draw their legs up to their chests and struggle as if they had to urinate. There is a possibility that your infant may arch their back, tighten their fists, and demonstrate other indications of distress (Healthdirect Australia, n.d.-a).

Tip

Colic pain may be lessened in some infants with gentle rocking, swaddling, and calming noises. In addition, making sure there is peace and quiet around your baby and experimenting with various feeding methods might be good.

Gas

Newborns with excess gas may show symptoms including crying, bloating, and frequent burping. Crying fits are a common side effect of gas pain. When you feel your baby's abdomen (stomach) between feedings, it should feel soft. There may be an issue if you notice any swelling or hardness. There is a possibility that your baby is experiencing constipation or gas. It could mean they have a gut problem if they haven't had a bowel movement in more than two days or if they are throwing up.

Tip

Babies benefit from mild stomach massage, being held upright after meals, and regular burping. If you're nursing, consider eliminating items that cause flatulence.

Reflux

When stomach acid flows back into the esophagus, it's called reflux. This can make your baby spit up or throw up. Your baby might cough or choke a little while they get used to eating simultaneously solid food daily. One sign that something could be wrong with their digestive system is if they cough or gag a lot when trying to eat. There is a chance that your baby will be uncomfortable after eating.

Tip

Your baby should be fed while sitting up, burped often, and kept elevated after each feeding. If your baby's acid reflux problems continue, you should see a doctor.

Jaundice

It's normal for the skin of newborn babies to seem somewhat yellow. This condition is known as jaundice. This condition manifests when a substance known as bilirubin accumulates in the infant's blood. It often manifests a few days after the baby is born and is common among infants. Cases of jaundice that are not severe are not harmful. The accumulation, however, might become problematic if it is allowed to reach an excessive level and therefore needs to be handled. The face is often the first part of the body to show signs of jaundice, followed by the chest and the belly, and then it moves on to the arms and the legs. As a secondary symptom, the whites of the eyes may sometimes become yellowish. Call your doctor immediately if you observe jaundice developing in your infant.

Tip

Either by nursing or formula, you should ensure your child is getting enough to drink. The condition often improves independently in mild episodes of jaundice; however, medical attention may be necessary in more severe cases.

Cow's Milk Protein Allergy

Some people with cow's milk protein allergy (CMPA) have eczema, stomachaches, and breathing difficulties. You'll need to closely monitor how your baby responds to various formulas and nursing methods.

Tip

If CMPA is suspected, the nursing mother should seek medical advice about using a unique formula or making dietary changes.

Respiratory Distress

A clogged nose is the most common cause of respiratory difficulties in infants. This is often easily fixed by utilizing saline nasal drops and a bulb syringe to remove the mucus. Your infant may also be suffering major respiratory issues if you notice the following symptoms:

- fast breathing (more than 60 breaths in one minute), but keep in mind that adults have slower breathing rates than infants. When this happens, the ribs protrude because the abdominal muscles in that area are constantly being compressed.

- nose enlargement

- grunting when inhaling

- Persistent blue coloring (*Recognizing Newborn Illnesses*, 2023)

You may need persistence, keen observation skills, and even expert assistance to overcome these typical obstacles. When in doubt, a parent should listen to their gut and look for outside help. We are in this together for your baby's happiness and health.

Chapter 7:

Parenting With Confidence

It is a great moment when parents hold their baby for the first time, but genuine parental confidence comes from a place more profound than that. Having the ability to recognize subtle cues, such as when they are hungry or when they want a diaper change, is what helps to establish confidence. The experience is like learning a coded language that only you and your child speak. The more attention and response parents pay to these indications, the more self-assured they grow in their ability to navigate parenthood's magnificent adventure.

Have you ever questioned the importance of parents expressing self-assurance? Even if you don't feel confident, you can still help your kid develop healthy self-esteem, correct? However, your self-assurance as a parent is vital not just for you but also for your children. Kids look up to their parents and try to emulate their actions. If you behave confidently in your decisions, it will provide a positive example for your child.

Self-assured babies are able to freely explore and learn since they know that a loved one will always be there for them. By responding to your baby's screams and other signals, such as scooping them up when they need comfort or retrieving the toy they're pointing to from the shelf, you can make your baby feel safe and secure by lavishing them with love and care. When you and your baby have a strong bond, your baby will gradually feel comfortable enough to venture out from you and explore the world around you. Your unwavering support will have gained their trust, which will instill confidence in your baby. As a new mother, it is very natural to not feel completely secure in your talents. However, the good news is that various methods can be used to gradually increase your expertise and confidence in yourself.

Bonding With Your Child

The intense emotional connection between a parent and their newborn is known as bonding. Because of this, parents feel an overwhelming need to adore and care for their newborn. As a means of bonding, caring for a newborn requires parents to pay close attention to their baby's screams and get up in the middle of the night to sate their growling hunger. Parents' strong bonds with their children set a good example for future close relationships and help babies feel safe and sound about their self-worth. How parents react to their babies' cues can also affect their social and mental growth. However, bonding is an ongoing process, not something that must occur immediately upon delivery or even within a specific time frame. Caring for a child daily often leads to a parent–child connection. When you see your kid smile for the first time, you may not even realize it's happening, but you'll be overwhelmed with excitement and love.

How Infants Form Bonds

As a new parent, it can take a while to get to know your baby and all the ways you can connect with them:

- Babies learn to communicate via touch when they react to skin-to-skin contact. As a bonus, this helps your baby develop normally and calms you and your little one.

- Close-range, meaningful conversation is facilitated by making direct eye contact.

- To keep up with moving things, babies may use their eyes.

- Your baby will attempt to mimic your every move and emotion from when they are tiny.

- Babies love to vocalize from the moment they first try to communicate, and prefer human sounds. Babies love to listen to stories about what you're doing, where you're taking them, and your own chats.

Among the many beautiful things about caring for a child is the opportunity to form a bond with your little one. Having loved ones who encourage you and believe in your parenting skills will make the transition to parenthood smoother. Because of this, it is advised by medical professionals that you have your infant remain in your hospital room. Taking care of a newborn may be a huge adjustment, but with the help of emotional support from hospital staff, you'll soon feel more prepared and capable (*Bonding With Your Baby*, n.d.).

Various Parent–Child Bonding Activities

Reading Together

- **Up to six months of age:**

    ○ Pick up some cuddly, brightly colored books with big illustrations.

    ○ Let your infant look at the pictures by holding the book near them.

    ○ Get their attention by making silly noises and pointing to visuals.

- **Six to twelve months:**

    ○ Share books that your child can engage with by adding noises and sensations.

    ○ Inspire your child to feel the pages and discover what's within.

    ○ To pique their interest, ask them basic questions regarding the visuals.

Baby Massage

- **From birth to three months old:**

    ○ In a warm room, work a fragrance-free baby oil into their skin slowly and gently.

    ○ Make gentle eye contact and speak soothingly to generate a relaxing mood.

- **Three to six months:**

    ○ Add additional interactive touches, such as light tapping of the fingers.

    ○ Keep an eye on their responses; you may want to ease off on the pressure if they seem uneasy.

    ○ Take advantage of this opportunity to establish a safe connection via physical contact.

Engaging in Sensory Experiences

- **Six to twelve months:**

    ○ Put together an essential sensory bin with nontoxic, roughly textured items.

    ○ Your infant will learn so much by exploring the world around them via touch.

    ○ Narrate events using descriptive terms to help with language development.

- **One year and beyond:**

    ○ Start with age-appropriate sensory activities, such as playing with playdough or finger paints.

- As you exhibit delight in their discoveries, encourage your child to use their senses.

- Participate in the play together, strengthening your bond via everyday experiences.

These tasks not only help your child grow emotionally and cognitively, but they also improve the bond between parent and child. It's essential to adapt the activities to your baby's needs and enjoy the process of growing up with them.

Establishing Routines and Schedules

"You need to get your baby on a schedule!" is a piece of advice that parents commonly hear. Maybe you're wondering when things will become more regular and predictable with your newborn since your routine is all over the place right now. Perhaps you need a timetable to ensure work punctuality or prepare your infant for their babysitter. Whatever the situation, you're probably considering how to institute regular sleep and wake times for your newborn.

The term "baby schedule" is understood somewhat differently by each individual. Some individuals see their baby schedules more as daily rituals or rhythms they perform with their infant. These routines often involve sleeping, feeding, and playing with their child. It is possible that some people have a habit of feeding their infant at the same time and in the same spot every morning, and that this eventually becomes their everyday routine. It is also possible for parents to begin to establish a nap routine for their infant, and, as a result, they begin to lay their child down for a nap at around the same time every day.

The most effective method for establishing a routine for your infant is to devote time to observing what your infant is doing at any given moment. You may find it useful to write down what you notice over a few days and then come up with a plan based on that information. It is essential to watch and discover how often your baby needs to take naps, how much sleep they need, and how many feedings they require. It is possible that some parents may wish to attempt to modify their baby's habits to better accommodate their family's existing lifestyle (Andruss, 2022).

Thinking back to the early days with my second child, it was like she had her little daily routine. At 9 p.m. sharp, she'd want her feed, and around 1 a.m., she'd wake up for a diaper change. After a cozy breastfeeding session at 4 a.m., she'd finally doze off until 6 a.m. Being a mom got pretty challenging in those first two months, but thankfully, my partner had my back. It made me realize that babies have unique quirks regarding eating and sleeping.

As time passed, my little one started adjusting to a schedule that worked for both of us. Now, as she grows, she's syncing up with my routine. It's a reminder that parenting is a learning curve, and with teamwork and understanding we can handle the ups and downs, turning challenges into shared moments of joy and connection.

We will now explore how a child's general health can be improved by establishing routines, especially regarding sleep and naps.

Benefits of Routines

Stability and Security

- Children get a feeling of security and comfort when they are exposed to a predictable environment, which is created by routines.

- Knowing what to anticipate helps establish a solid basis for your mental well-being.

Promoting Self-Care

- The ability to carve out specific time for self-care is made possible for parents by establishing routines.

- Parents have the ability to prioritize their well-being by establishing routines, which might include activities like quiet meditation or the pursuit of personal hobbies.

Enhancing Confidence

- Children develop a sense of self-assurance when exposed to consistent routines, which also serve as a framework to comprehend and manage their day-to-day lives.

- If you are a parent, having a planned routine may help relieve stress and give you a feeling of control over the activities you have to do each day.

Practical Tips for Establishing Routines

Sleeping/Naps

- Make a routine that will help you relax before going to bed, such as reading or listening to soft music.

- Maintaining a regular schedule for a child's nap and sleep hours benefits the child's mental clock.

Meal Planning

- The week's meals should be planned ahead, considering the family's nutritional requirements and tastes.

- It is essential to designate specific mealtimes to foster a shared and pleasurable experience for the family.

Task Allocation

- Clearly outline the roles that each family member is responsible for, such as cooking.

- Establishing a plan for home duties is essential to ensure that responsibilities are distributed fairly.

Flexibility Within the Routine

- Even though routines provide structure, they should also leave space for flexibility to accept unforeseen developments.

- Adapt your routines to accommodate the changing dynamics of the household as your children grow.

When routines are incorporated into everyday life, it creates a more structured and peaceful atmosphere, which beneficially affects children and parents. This is because routines contribute significantly to a family's general well-being and efficiency, making the demands of busy lifestyles more bearable. Routines provide several benefits, including the certainty of regular sleep patterns and the convenience of food preparation.

Being Present

The idea of "being present" is to enjoy the time spent with your children fully, including the moments when you laugh together, get embraces out of the blue, or convert a challenging situation into an opportunity for growth. We have all heard stories from our parents that show how quickly time passed when we were kids. The days may seem long, but the years are short. The truth, however, is that you don't have to savor every moment. There will inevitably be highs and lows as a parent.

The easy ways to be more present include putting phones aside on essential occasions, breathing deeply to maintain awareness, and paying close attention when you're with your children. The goal is to practice mindfulness, live in the now without judging or critiquing, and relax. Being a parent is a wild and wonderful adventure; being present is about embracing the ride and being gentle with ourselves.

Being fully present is a notion that I think is crucial for our infants and, significantly, us to be able to comprehend what is happening in their developing brains; therefore, I wanted to start a discussion about it. Understanding how and why to live in the now has many advantages. When I say we should be present at certain times with our newborns, I mean it on all levels: cerebral, emotional, and spiritual. According to what I have learned, being physically present with a baby is one of the most precious things a parent can provide them. My experience in the sector has led me to believe this to be true. Being present is like giving our infants a gift—and it's not easy for us to pull it off, you know? In the words of Thich Nhat Hahn, "Life can be found only in the present moment. The past is gone. The future is not here yet, and if we do not return to ourselves in the present moment, we cannot be in touch with life" (Hanh, n.d.).

At this point, it is essential to realize that, even though it may seem challenging, you have to make every effort to be mentally, physically, and spiritually present as often as possible. In all honesty, it is essential for your child's growth and development, and it provides a multitude of advantages for both you and your child.

Now I will explain what I mean when someone is physically, emotionally, and spiritually present.

Being Physically Present With Your Baby

One of the best ways to help your baby grow and develop is to be physically there for them. All of these methods allow for the physical presence of parents:

- direct skin contact

- tummy time

- gentle massages

- kissing and hugging

- floor playtime

- reading together

- singing and talking

- answering cues

Remember, being physically present goes beyond being in the same room. Actively engage with your infant, react to their needs, and create moments of connection to build a loving bond.

Being Mentally Present With Your Baby

Maintaining a mental presence in the face of a seemingly endless stream of stimuli may be challenging. However, being present gives your infant the chance to engage in conversation and form connections. Plus, you get to see life through their eyes:

- Find joy in routine activities like bath time, diaper changes, and bedtime.

- Explain your actions and emotions to your infant. This introduces them to language and connects them to your world.

- Focus on your baby's coos, screams, and babbles to practice reflective listening, make eye contact and smile at your infant, and engage with your infant during playtime.

Being mentally present means connecting with your child, noticing their needs, and enjoying each day's unique experiences.

Being Spiritually Present With Your Baby

Spiritual presence provides hope, pleasure, and amazement to your child's life. A more detailed grasp of their growth is also gained. This way, we can see them as humans with unlimited potential.

- Create a peaceful environment for your infant. Dim lighting, calm music, or natural noises can create a relaxing mood.

- Use basic spiritual practices like a quick prayer, thankfulness, or bedtime blessings.

Spiritual presence is individualized and varies by belief (*3 Amazing Ways to Be Present With Your Baby*, 2021).

Avoiding Comparisons

As parents, it is essential that you avoid comparing your children to those of other families. Every child is unique and develops at their own pace regardless of age. You need to rejoice in the qualities that make your children unique. Because social media may only highlight the positive aspects of parenting, you must restrict the time you spend looking at it. Instead of focusing on what your kids cannot do, concentrate on what they excel in. Conversations with other parents about your experiences may be beneficial; nevertheless, it is essential to remember that every family is different. A happy family is one in which each member can trust their unique parenting style and recognize and appreciate their child's qualities, even the more insignificant ones.

You should make it a priority to constantly want to bring value to your connection with your infant, and comparing your child to others may have a detrimental impact on your confidence in both yourself and your baby.

The Risks of Comparing Your Child to Others

Missing Milestones

You might overlook your baby's milestones by focusing on their shortcomings. Be watchful of your baby's progress. Comparing your infant to others emphasizes what they can't accomplish rather than what they can. Your baby will reach huge and tiny milestones and, no matter the size, a milestone is a milestone!

Having Doubts

When you compare yourself to other moms, you start to doubt yourself and lose faith in yourself. Maybe another child reached a milestone before yours, but that doesn't mean you failed. You didn't do anything wrong. It also doesn't mean that the other child's mother is doing anything different from what you are doing.

Missing Moments

You may miss precious bonding moments by wishing your infant would do something else. Waiting for your child to try something new might prevent lovely bonding moments like the one above. Be in a moment!

Being Overwhelmed by Stress

Thinking that your child is falling behind might potentially cause you to worry more than you already are. When you hear that another kid is doing something your baby is not yet doing, it is tempting to conclude that your baby is falling behind other children. Without a doubt, I've been there!

Feeling Discouraged

You may be discouraged, making it more challenging to have a healthy connection with your child. We may not always be aware of this, but when we are angry, disappointed, or unhappy, we tend to take it out on our children in the most peculiar ways. It is possible to grow to concentrate on the bad, the "things my baby isn't doing yet," and entirely dismiss what our baby is accomplishing. Pay attention to the good (Brianna, 2020)!

To foster your child's development, establish a nurturing atmosphere. Avoiding comparisons and embracing your family's unique path makes parenting healthier and more satisfying.

Chapter 8:

Returning to Work

Returning to work after all the fun and chaos of giving birth is challenging. New moms have to carefully balance the responsibilites of their jobs with the deep joys and challenges of being a parent. To make this change go smoothly, you must be careful about balancing your work goals and the rewarding role of motherhood.

Going back to work after having a child can be a big step. As this time gets closer, you might feel many different things. You might be scared to return to work or feel bad about leaving your child with someone else. On the other hand, you could be thrilled about the possibility of going back to work and having the opportunity to catch up with your regular coworkers. Resuming employment is a personal choice. Many factors might come into play here, such as your job situation, family dynamics, financial situation, and your child's adaptability to new situations. Several aspects should be considered before making the decision. Resuming work after giving birth is a personal decision for each new mother, and, like many other parts of pregnancy and the postpartum period, there is no universally accepted schedule. Although some mothers take a full year off work after giving birth, others return to work as soon as a few weeks have passed.

Mothers may need help to return to work immediately after maternity leave. A new parent's life is in entire upheaval, and you're already feeling the pinch of having to go back to work. Don't worry—we'll help. To make this change more accessible and help you find a balance between your job and family life, let's talk about some concrete steps you can take.

Planning for Childcare

Planning for childcare is essential for new parents who are returning to work or for parents who need extra help taking care of their young ones. In the beginning, being a parent can feel like balancing everything, and ensuring your child has a safe and caring place to live takes a lot of thought and planning. As parents, we are responsible for ensuring our children are well-prepared for this change by securing suitable childcare. You deserve to be able to relax when you're away from your child, and finding a reliable childcare provider is a big part of that. Working parents will have a wide range of childcare alternatives depending on location, family income, and company flexibility.

Researching and Visiting Potential Childcare Options

Early planning means looking into and seeing different childcare choices before you need them. This can include looking into daycare centers, babysitters who come to your house, or family members who are ready to help. Daycare centers offer social contact, while home-based care provides more individualized care. Each choice has its own pros and cons.

Considering Cost and Availability

Caregiving services should be considered in terms of availability and cost. Please determine how much the chosen arrangement will cost and ensure it fits your budget. Also, think about how many spots are available in daycares or how flexible the schedules of in-home workers are. Parents often choose from the following options when it comes to childcare.

Daycare

Make sure to talk to a lot of nearby childcare providers before choosing the one that fits your family's needs the best. This is true whether you choose an approved in-home provider or a daycare center. When parents look for daycares, they often talk about the following things:

- Does this daycare provider have a license?

- Is it near or easy to get to from home, my workplace or the job of my partner?

- How much does this place and/or the sitter charge each week or month?

- Are there online reviews I can read, or do they have links I can check out?

- In total, how many kids are cared for? How many are in each classroom? How many babysitters are there, and how many kids do they take care of?

Parents should plan to visit any daycares they are interested in before making a reservation for childcare. Some daycares only take a certain number of babies, and others may have a waiting list for new kids. This is especially true if you live in an area with few daycares. Most of the time, it's best to start looking into babysitting choices for working parents and planning when you'll return to work after maternity leave before you give birth. This way, your family will be ready.

A private caregiver is often responsible for a child's well-being, so most parents send their children to daycare. This includes feeding and entertaining your child, and keeping them safe. Private caregivers may have backgrounds ranging from basic childcare training to advanced early childhood education. Private caregivers may provide more flexible scheduling and duties. They customize daycare to family requirements. Private caregivers give each child their full attention and customize activities and learning.

Private Caregiver or Nanny

Many mothers hire a private caregiver for their children to provide them with a more individualized and adaptable caring arrangement. As a one-on-one service, private nannies give each kid their full attention, ensuring they are in a setting that fits their nature and stage of growth. Private care is especially appealing because it allows families to change plans and caring styles to fit their needs. This one-on-one care builds a strong bond between the caretaker and the child, making the child feel safe and trusting. Some moms also like that private nannies can offer a more flexible and personalized approach, ensuring the child's well-being is at the center of their parenting journey. Private caregivers, like nannies, are expensive but usually come to your house (*Working Moms*, n.d.).

In some families, the caregiver may be your spouse, your parents, or other family member or friend. This gives caregivers some flexibility and peace of mind, but they should have backup plans in case the caregiver becomes ill, has an emergency, or travel sout of town.

Tips for Finding Trustworthy Childcare Providers

Finding excellent childcare may be challenging for parents. There are many things to look for and ask at a childcare center. Can you tell whether your child would be happy there? Will they accommodate your child? Are there progress reports for your child? What if your child dislikes it? Every choice has pros and cons, so evaluating each one and getting as much information as possible is necessary. The following advice will assist you:

- Check childcare providers' safety. This includes safe spaces, age-appropriate toys, and emergency procedures.

- Ask caregivers about their credentials. Child development and first aid training are valuable.

- Ask other parents who have utilized daycare for recommendations. Their experiences may provide insights.

- Visit childcare facilities during operating hours to observe daily routines and interactions. Watch how in-home professionals interact with youngsters.

Finally, childcare planning takes time, so allow for it. Better daycare choices are available if you start early (Park Academy Childcare, 2022).

FAQs for Daycare Center Tours

- What is the staff-to-child ratio, and how does the center ensure individualized attention?

- Can you share the safety measures in place, including emergency procedures and childproofing?

- What daily activities are provided, and how are they tailored to different age groups?

- How are meals handled, and can accommodations be made for special dietary needs?

- How does the center involve parents in their child's daily experiences, and what communication channels are in place?

- What are the center's policies regarding sick children? How do you handle illnesses, and what measures are taken to prevent the spread of infections?

- Can you provide information on the training and qualifications of the staff? How do you ensure that the caregivers are well-prepared to handle various situations?

- How are outdoor play areas designed for safety, and how often do children get outdoor playtime? What safety measures are in place during outdoor activities?

- What emergency procedures are in place? How often are emergency drills conducted, and how are parents informed about the outcomes?

- How does the center handle the transition period for new children? Are there specific strategies to help children adjust to the new environment?

- How does the center handle separation anxiety in young children? Are specific routines or activities in place to ease the transition between drop-off and pick-up?

- What is the center's approach to discipline? How are behavioral issues addressed, and what strategies are used to promote positive behavior?

- How does the center accommodate children with special needs? Are there specific programs or resources in place to support diverse learning requirements?

- Can you provide examples of the daily learning and developmental activities planned for different age groups? How are these activities tailored to each child's developmental stage?

- What backup plans are in place if a caregiver is absent? How does the center ensure continuity of care in such situations?

- Are there opportunities for parents to get involved in the center's activities or events? How does the center encourage parent participation in the child's learning journey?

These questions on your childcare facility tour checklist will help you acquire all the information you need to judge the center's appropriateness for your child.

Managing Time and Priorities

One of the most common struggles for new mothers is finding a balance between their careers and being a parent. The ability to effectively manage your time and establish priorities compatible with your work and personal life is crucial to success. Striking the balance between being too rigid and too flexible is a challenging feat. Many mothers share the same sentiments when they say, "I am unable to spend quality time with my infants." And those are the moments when the guilt trips we experience as working mothers begin.

Life is hard when balancing work, home, family, and, most importantly, being a parent. For working moms, setting boundaries is one of the most valuable things they can do.

Setting Boundaries

Clear boundaries between work and personal time can help you maintain balance. Ensure your family and coworkers know these limits by letting them know when you're available and when you need focused, undivided time for work or family duties. As a working mom, you must learn to make time for yourself and your daily tasks. Believe me, I know. You'll feel better soon enough after making a few changes here and there.

Learning to Delegate Tasks

Being a supermom doesn't mean you have to do everything by yourself. Mastering the art of delegation is a potent tactic that can be used in every setting. Find things that can be divided up or handed off to someone else, whether at work or at home. New mothers can free up time and energy to concentrate on what matters when they delegate tasks to others.

Recognizing the Need for Flexibility

Adaptability is essential for new mothers to manage their time effectively. Recognizing the need to adjust plans is crucial when dealing with the unpredictability of life with a baby. Please keep an open mind as you may need to change your professional and personal schedules on a dime when you least anticipate it.

Simplifying Your Meal Plans

Organizing meals as a mother is a beautiful responsibility. When you have kids around, planning meals, grocery shopping, and cooking is hard work. If you have a plan for the week, you'll succeed in failing miserably as the unexpected will undoubtedly occur. Consider using a calendar that includes a menu to simplify your weekdays. Just 30 minutes will give you plenty of time to decide what to eat and list everything you need from the grocery store.

Scheduling Your Household Chores

Juggling job and domestic responsibilities requires a lot of physical stamina for working mothers. Instead of doing little tasks every day, choose one day and accomplish everything at once. For instance, designate a weekday to handle things like ironing, laundry, or physical food shopping. Instead of doing everything every day, set aside a specific day to do certain duties.

Establishing Fixed Working Hours

Ask yourself if you are really ready to take on new tasks before you do so. Make sure that your boss and you both agree on what your work hours will be. There will always be responsibilities and projects at work, so make sure that standards have not changed.

Setting Achievable Daily Goals

It is pointless to have an overly ambitious list of things to accomplish. If you know you will not be able to complete the duties you have written down, what is the use of making that list? Your goal should not be to become a superhero, since you are not one. Ensure that your daily objectives are attainable and within your reach. Always remember that you can always do more if you have the time.

Remembering to Have Some Fun!

Stressed people can't do anything. It would help if you took a break to avoid burnout at work and home. Plan holidays, long weekends, and family parties to stay stable and happy (WOW Parenting, 2019).

My number one advice for working mothers is to always be ready. How well you plan doesn't matter; something will always go wrong. For example, the sports practice might get canceled, your child might have a temper tantrum at the last minute, and so on. The most important thing is to be ready to drop your plans and go with the flow.

Know your rights before you go back to work. The Fair Labor Standards Act (FLSA) says that if you are breastfeeding, your boss must make certain simple adjustments. The PUMP for Nursing Mothers Act (the "PUMP Act") says that all nursing moms must have "a place, other than a bathroom, that is shielded from view to express breast milk while at work." You have this right for up to a year after your child's birth. Whether you are paid by the hour or the month, your employer must follow this rule (Squillace, 2023).

For busy moms who are having a hard time with nursing, knowing how to pump or do combi feeding during the workday is essential. It is necessary to know about the legal rights that moms have to ensure they have the time and place to pump if they want to. Setting up a regular time to pump, talking to your managers about specific needs, and finding a quiet and comfy place to pump can all help nursing fit more easily into your workday.

Recognizing the Significance of Self-Care

Taking care of yourself is even more necessary when balancing work and being a mom. This means recognizing your needs, taking breaks when needed, and making time to relax. In the next chapter, we'll talk more about how important it is for working moms to take care of themselves, focusing on how a healthy mom makes both mom and baby healthier.

Maintaining Personal Fulfillment and Identity

Keeping your personality and sense of satisfaction is essential outside of being a mother. Many new moms feel better and more confident when they pursue hobbies, interests, or work goals separate from their role as moms. Not only do these activities make you happier, but they also make your family more substantial as a whole. Combining new parenthood and work duties requires time management, limits, and flexibility. New parents can gracefully handle this challenging but rewarding journey by using these tactics.

Building a Support Network

Everyone has heard the expression "it takes a village" at some point. But as moms today, we're expected to do everything, and it can be hard to get help when needed. And even for those lucky moms who get a lot of help initially, the help decreases a lot after the first year. You may have already seen this. It's possible that your moms' group has broken up, friends have stopped dropping by as often, or everyone you know has gone back to work.

Additionally, one of the sad truths about being a mom today is that even though we've never been more connected (thanks to things like social media), we've never felt less linked as people. Moms need a village, which means a group of people to help them.

You need a group of people and services that share your beliefs, are there for you through good times and bad, and help you find peace in your daily life. Being a mother is hard. You were never meant to do it by yourself. You need to build your town, even if it doesn't look quite how you thought it would.

Importance of Seeking Support

Working and caring for family duties simultaneously is hard for everyone. Asking for help is not a sign of weakness; it's a recognition of how complex modern parenting is. Support networks can provide comfort, direction, and understanding when you feel unsure or overwhelmed.

This support network is open to all parents because it knows that the problems stay-at-home moms face are just as acute as those of working moms. Your network will incorporate a lot of different situations and events, building a sense of community that goes beyond the usual lines between these jobs.

Guidance on Building a Support Network

Create Time and Space for Nurturing Your Relationship at Home

We all love our homes. Your partner is the one person you should always be able to count on. Your relationship with your partner was essential to you before you had a child. You'd go on dates and talk about your hopes and goals and your days. You'd be there for each other no matter what. Some of these connections break down for many couples after they have kids. You barely have time to do everything you need to, let alone work on your relationship. You both look and feel tired, stressed, and maybe even a little alone.

Make sure you and your partner have regular time to talk. Do not use your phones or watch TV during this time. Talk about how you both feel over a cup of coffee or a glass of wine. Try to see things from the other person's point of view without judging. This may be hard because you might feel you deserve to be heard the most. But try anyway. It doesn't need to be a fancy meal or night out. It's an average time to check in with each other. This easy job will improve your relationship, and if you talk to each other well, you should be able to agree on everything. Talk freely about your duties and work together to find ways to balance work and home life.

Building and Nurturing Your Inner Circle

Use the help of family and friends who live nearby. Getting help from people close to you can make things easier, whether it's about childcare or helpful advice. This group of people is the small group you talk to often and can be fully honest with. Don't be hard on yourself if you don't have this yet—this is something a lot of women experience after having kids. One reason might be that none of their friends have kids, so they're suddenly living a very different life from the ones their friends can relate to. Look for other moms who work in your area or at work. Sharing stories, advice, and problems with people going through the same things builds understanding and strength. Look into parenting groups or playdate communities in your area. Getting in touch with local parents can help you share stories and find tools in your area. Use the vast amount of information available in online parenting groups—blogs, social media groups, and forums provide a virtual place to share tips, ask questions, and get help from a larger community.

Creating and Nurturing Your Outer Circle

The outside world, where we spend a lot of time, is the last step in forming your community. In a real sense, this could mean your neighborhood, the coffee shop, the school, or even your friends and family. Finding people and places that make you feel safe, happy, and stable is essential. That's the simple part. The hardest part of your outside group is how you use social media. Look through your social media feeds with a plan. Choose who to follow and what posts to see.

Home life, inner and outer groups, and the balance between them will differ for everyone. It's essential to find the balance that works for you. Work on improving one area at a time until you find a good blend if you need to improve your network (*3 Ways to Build a Support Network as a Mother*, n.d.).

Chapter 9:

Self-Care and Wellness for Mothers

Some mothers may feel stressed by being a mom and may put their families' needs before their own. Other moms try to find a middle ground between their own health and their children's health since self-care can significantly influence one's emotional, mental, and physical well-being. Learning how to properly practice self-care may be essential to being a mother. In addition to the many advantages that this ability will bring into your life, you may also be able to acquire healthy coping methods with the assistance of someone with expertise.

When my newest baby arrived, mornings were like a crazy puzzle. I had to get my two older kids ready for daycare and ensure my husband had breakfast before work. The kitchen was a mess by the time he left with the kids. Left alone with my newborn, I faced a mountain of work. After finishing everything, I wanted to nap or do other things before my older kids came back. It was stressful, and finding time for myself seemed an impossible task. But I knew deep down that taking care of myself was super important. Even though I wasn't a superhero like Wonder Woman, I realized taking a break and looking after myself was okay. So, I embraced the messy kitchen and the stress, understanding that a mom who cares for herself can better care for her family. Self-care isn't selfish and you shouldn't feel guilty about prioritizing your needs. No self-care routine is perfect. Finding quiet time to reflect is all that's needed. The first step in practicing self-care is to develop a sense of curiosity. An important reason why self-care is essential is that it allows you to concentrate on yourself rather than being consumed by other factors like work, family, or relationships.

The advantages of self-care for moms are as follows:

- lower chance of getting health problems like heart disease in the future

- more time to spend on making and keeping human connections

- strengthens how you see yourself

- more self-esteem

You can protect your mental health by practicing self-care. Taking care of yourself gives you valuable skills for dealing with stress. It can also help you deal with sadness and worry better if you are already experiencing these emotions (BetterHelp Editorial Team, 2023).

Managing Stress

New mothers often experience a flurry of stress due to the combination of the pleasures and difficulties that come with early parenting. Recognizing the significance of effectively managing this stress is not only an act of self-care but also an essential step in ensuring the mother's well-being and a good quality of life for her family. Practical relaxation methods may be helpful tools when caring for a newborn and managing the stresses of returning to work and the inevitable sleep loss. Stress in the first few years of motherhood can be anticipated and controlled in many ways. If you or a loved one are a new parent coping with the stresses of the transition, here are some tactics that have helped other new parents manage.

Be Aware of Your Expectations

As a parent, you may find that your actual situation differs from your imagined ideal. Many of your ideas and hopes about how happy being a parent would make you will have been shaped in some way by ads, magazines, books, and talking to friends and family about their own experiences. Societal expectations of motherhood are so high, and the experience seems so great, that it may be hard to confess that you are struggling.

Be ready for many scenarios, including times when you struggle and don't understand what's happening because you are still learning a lot. It is natural to have bad days; some people may have worse days than others. As a new parent, you are not alone in feeling stressed.

Consider Exercise for Stress Release

Getting some exercise can help with both mental and physical stress. Relaxing your muscles, taking a break, or going to a different place can all help your body release feel-good chemicals called endorphins. It can also help you focus on something else. Making time for awareness activities can help new moms find their center amid all the chaos. An essential mindfulness practice, such as deep breathing, guided meditation, or awareness of one's immediate environment, may profoundly affect your emotional and mental well-being.

Don't Expect Too Much of Yourself

There are always more duties to perform, but does it matter if not everything gets done or isn't perfect? Remember to relish the pleasant times. Give yourself some time. Take it easy, unwind, and relax; you deserve it.

Stop Comparing Yourself to Others

Stop comparing yourself to other people. No two people's situations are the same. It's not a competition; nobody comes out on top. Stand by yourself.

Reach Out and Connect With Friends, Family, and Professionals

Stop trying to solve problems yourself and ask for help. Get in touch with your support network. If you're feeling lonely or alone, all it takes is a quick phone call or online chat to connect with someone and get some much-needed perspective. Another option is to contact one of the many expert helplines available. Seek assistance without hesitation or embarrassment. Some may find this challenging, but many around you will welcome the chance to pitch in and provide a hand.

Be Aware of How Much Stress You Are Under and How Long You Have Felt This Way

Feelings of stress are normal; nevertheless, they may become distressing and raise the risk of PPD, anxiety, and other mental health issues if they persist for long periods instead of passing quickly. Set your infant down in a secure area (like their crib) and give yourself a break. You can lessen anxious feelings by practicing deep breathing, listening to music, or chatting with someone. When things become challenging, it's common for parents to feel this way. It will help if you gave yourself time to collect your thoughts and realize that this will pass (*Managing Stress in Early Parenthood*, n.d.).

It's important to know what these disorders are and how to recognize their symptoms to ensure you get good care when you need it. An essential part of managing stress is making sure you get enough sleep and take care of yourself. One way to strengthen your ability to bounce back from setbacks is to make time for rest and relaxation a regular part of one's routine.

Exercise and Physical Activity

We've already talked about how important exercise and physical activity are, so let's go into more detail about how regular physical activity after giving birth can make a huge difference in a woman's health and happiness, with effects far beyond the first few weeks of healing. As the body heals, doing safe and effective workouts helps with physical healing and improves mental health. This is called a "holistic" approach to postpartum fitness. Regular exercise after giving birth can:

- help you lose weight if you also cut back on calories

- strengthen your heart and lungs

- tone and strengthen your abs

- bring more energy to you

For me, the best exercise is running after my toddler—the original HIIT workout!

Benefits of Exercise

- Regular exercise aids postpartum muscle and tissue healing. Strength, flexibility, and cardiovascular health may also improve.

- Exercise boosts mood. Exercise releases endorphins, which reduce postpartum blues and promote well-being.

- Regular exercise improves sleep. A steady exercise plan may help new parents with sleep deprivation sleep better.

- Exercise is a powerful stress reducer.

Safe and Effective Postpartum Exercises

Yoga is a tremendous postpartum workout for all fitness levels. Gentle stretching, core strengthening, and relaxation are its main objectives. Yoga sessions for postpartum women sometimes include modifications

Walking is a low-impact, easily accessible kind of exercise that can be tailored to the specific fitness level of the person. It gives you fresh air to breathe and offers a light cardiovascular workout that may be readily included in various daily routines.

Strength training can be advantageous if it is undertaken in a moderate manner to facilitate postpartum healing. It helps in regaining muscular strength and can be adapted to the specific fitness levels of each person. To guarantee healthy development, it is best to begin with exercises that use your body weight and then progressively include modest weights (*Exercise During Pregnancy*, n.d.).

Recommendations for Safe Postpartum Exercise

Before beginning any postpartum fitness routine, it is necessary to discuss the matter with a healthcare expert. They can give individualized guidance that takes into account the individual's health as well as any particular concerns associated with their birth experience. It would help to start with light activities and progressively increase the intensity as your body recovers. Initially, it would help if you steer clear of high-impact activities and instead concentrate on building a solid foundation before beginning more intense workouts. Pay attention to keeping a healthy posture when you are exercising. This is of utmost significance as the body returns to normal after giving birth. Effective workouts that limit the risk of injury are those that are performed with proper alignment. New mothers can start the path to physical and emotional wellness by engaging in safe and effective postpartum workouts, including walking, yoga, and strength training.

Embracing Body Positivity

It can be challenging for women to love their bodies, especially after giving birth and during the time afterward. Body shaming after giving birth is a common problem that many new moms have to deal with. It adds extra stress and worry to a time that is already hard. Society often puts too much pressure on women to quickly "bounce back" to the bodies that they had before they got pregnant. Being a mom means our bodies have been stretched beyond and back; we don't always "bounce back," and things may be a bit wigglier and jigglier after creating a tiny human inside us. Some days, looking in the mirror and loving our skin can be challenging. This can make women question themselves and feel like they're not good enough. We need to change the narrative and start loving ourselves and our bodies.

Modern moms are told all the time that diets will help them "fix" their bodies. Many moms base their beliefs on what they see in ads, but that's not how it is to be a mom. We're starting to come out of the fantasy world where our self-worth is set by someone else who makes money from our fears. You can uncover this truth by filtering out the diet industry's multibillion-dollar buzz. If we tried to undo the changes in our bodies, we would have to erase every moment and the path that led us to our children. After having a baby, your body changes to show that this beautiful process has occurred. Why do you need to fix it right away? Rest up and pay attention to your body. You are not a model or a celebrity. Instead, work on having a good attitude about your body as a mother and celebrate the remarkable changes you have experienced and are still going through.

First and foremost, you should be aware of the physical changes after giving birth. A woman's body goes through many changes throughout pregnancy and giving birth. Gaining weight, stretch marks, sagging skin, and changes to the size and form of the breasts are all examples of these changes. It's important to acknowledge that these changes are lovely and standard for being a mother.

Recognizing the adverse effects of body shaming is the first step in effectively combatting it, which brings us to the second key factor. When we are subjected to body shaming, whether it originates from outside sources or from inside ourselves, it has a significant influence on our sense of belonging and our general health and happiness.

Strategies to Promote Self-Esteem and a Positive Body Image

While some mothers welcome the physical and emotional changes that accompany pregnancy and childbirth, many women find that these experiences have a profoundly detrimental impact on their perception of self-identity. Apart from that, women who experience body image dissatisfaction are four times as likely to have perinatal depression (Horsager-Boehrer, 2022). Embrace your changing self-image after delivery with the following strategies for a pleasant and robust experience.

Enjoy the Miracle of Life

The time during pregnancy and after giving birth is impressive and shows how strong and resilient the female body is. Accept that your body is making a new life and caring for it. Know that every change, even ones you can't see, is a sign of the beauty of motherhood and parenting.

Accept Your Transformation

Your body will change independently as your baby grows. Accept your postpartum pooch, bigger breasts, and curvier body. Instead of focusing on what you think is wrong with your body, see these changes as beautiful and unique signs of being a mother. Identify and fight against social norms that aren't reasonable. Know that every woman's journey after giving birth is different, and it's not fair or reasonable to compare yourself to a perfect picture.

Focus on Health and Inner Strength

Instead of focusing on your appearance, put your inner power and health first. Do good things for your body and mind, like meditation, light exercise, and postnatal yoga. Self-care is essential for keeping your body and mind healthy.

Surround Yourself With Positive People

Get help from family, friends, and other women who have children and know what it's like to go through childbirth and body changes. Having positive people around you can lift your mood and help you remember that you are not alone in what you are going through.

Accept the Emotional Roller Coaster

During motherhood, hormones can make you feel a range of emotions, from happiness to occasional worry or mood swings. Remember that these feelings are normal and a part of the journey. Don't judge yourself as you feel and talk about your feelings.

Record Your Journey

Take pictures or write in a book to remember your pregnancy. Taking pictures of your changing body and thoughts while expecting a child can help you remember this life-changing time with love and respect.

Dress to Look Good and Feel Good

As your body changes, buy stylish motherhood clothes that make you feel good about yourself. It can help your confidence and self-image to wear clothes that fit well and look good on your changed body.

Talk With Your Partner

Talk to your partner honestly about how you're feeling while being a mom. Your partner's support and understanding can help you feel better about yourself during this time.

Self-Compassion Is Essential

Self-compassion means being kind to yourself. Don't compare yourself to other people or have unrealistic standards of yourself. Don't forget that each pregnancy is different, but everyone's is beautiful (*Pregnancy and Body Changes*, n.d.).

Nutrition and Exercise as Forms of Self-Regulation

It is essential to see diet and exercise as tools for self-regulation instead of ways to control your weight. Resisting outside pressures and take a balanced approach that supports your general health and well-being. Focus on feeling strong and healthy.

In the end, the time after giving birth is a time to embrace body positivity and self-love. Mothers can endure this challenging time with strength by questioning social norms, practicing self-compassion, and putting total self-care first. They can also enjoy the fantastic journey their bodies have been on.

Chapter 10:

Beyond the Fourth Trimester

As a mother, the time after the fourth trimester is a new beginning full of joy and many questions. After the joys of pregnancy and the life-changing time after giving birth, the next stage brings new challenges and tasks that change how family life works. The weeks rapidly turn into months; before you know it, your infant is six months old. We, as mothers, need to be ready to update our infant menus as we begin offering solid foods to our children when they reach the six-month mark. It is like opening a little door to a whole new gastronomic cosmos for your young one; it is messy, without a doubt, but it is very satisfying!

You also need to remember to sleep. Let's be honest—it's a hot topic. We'll explore how to cope with those interrupted zzzs. Because, let's face it, moms need their beauty sleep too (and maybe a bit more coffee) And then there is the delicate art of returning to work after a break. Keeping up with the responsibilities of your profession, maintaining your home, cultivating connections, taking care of yourself, and caring for your developing child all at the same time seems like a lot. Do not be concerned; we are here to assist you in discovering your natural flow. Your duty as a parent is comparable to that of a superhero with a wide range of abilities, including the ability to nurture, lead, supply, and offer assistance in general. You're doing a fantastic job, even if it's a little overwhelming.

We are here to cheer you on, celebrate the successes, conquer the problems, and delight in the ever-evolving tapestry of family life. Life beyond the fourth trimester is like a new adventure every day, and we are here to help you make the most of it.

In many cases, women who suffer from PPD report feeling less attached to their children. It is not uncommon to have feelings of numbness, worthlessness, or hopelessness. A lot of women experience mood swings, anger, or crying often. Although some people have problems falling asleep, others seem to have difficulty getting out of bed. So, let's discuss how mothers can be strong in the long run, both physically and mentally.

Long-Term Physical and Emotional Well-Being

When you hear the term "healthy," what thoughts come to mind? A physically fit person is probably the first thing that comes to mind. The mental components of health often don't immediately occur to us when it comes to health, as we have been taught to focus on the physical parts of health.

However, it is just as crucial to prioritize your mental health as it is to prioritize your physical health, particularly after you have given birth. It is essential to create room in your life for mental well-being, and here are some recommendations that will help you do just that.

Why is your mental health so important? And what exactly is mental health? Our emotional, psychological, and social well-being are all components of our mental health, as stated by the Centers for Disease Control and Prevention (n.d.-a). This has an impact on how we think, feel, and behave. Also, it helps define how we deal with stress, interact with other people, and choose to make good decisions.

Mental health is considered one of the "four pillars of health." If your mind, body, and spirit were built into a home, these four components would be a solid foundation:

- **Nutrition:** In terms of nutrition, anything you put into your body will affect your performance.

- **Activity:** Physical activity, including exercise and movement, benefits how your body operates.

- **Sleep:** When you get enough quality sleep, it can have a significant impact on both your health and your emotions. The inability to get enough sleep may have a substantial effect on your view of the world, as well as on your health, in both the short and long term.

- **Mental health:** Your ability to deal with stress and worry and your resilience are all characteristics that fall under the mental health category.

When compared to the other three pillars, mental health is often overlooked, even though it plays a significant role in day-to-day living. However, paying attention to all four is essential to achieve the highest possible pleasure and well-being.

This is particularly true for moms. A weaker immune system, persistent discomfort, changes in weight, and other adverse physical changes may be the result of neglecting your mental health, which can also lead to difficulties in connecting with your child, strained relationships, and other adverse outcomes. If you choose to disregard your emotions, you may be increasing the likelihood of experiencing stress, despair, anxiety, and burnout. These are indeed issues you may face at any time, but during the postpartum period they are of the most immense significance (Maas, 2023).

Tips for Long-Term Health After the Postpartum Period

- Self-care methods learned early on are essential for well-being and resilience.

- Regular exercise is a lifetime commitment to health. Postpartum-friendly activities such as yoga and customized fitness regimens boost emotional and physical health.

- Parenthood brings continual stress. Manage it well.

- Nurturing social bonds is timeless. Making time for meaningful relationships with friends, family, and other parents, building a support system that will only grow more important.

- Conversations about mental health don't just happen after giving birth. Try to share your feelings with your loved ones.

Addressing Lingering Concerns

- **Pelvic floor health:** Maintaining a healthy pelvic floor goes well beyond the time immediately after giving birth. The key to avoiding and dealing with problems is consistent exercise and advice from healthcare experts.

- **Physical pain or discomfort:** Do not ignore any persistent pain or discomfort. It's best to see a healthcare expert or specialist to have physical issues handled quickly and thoroughly.

- **Mental health support:** A proactive measure to take if your emotional issues continue is to seek out mental health specialists. Consistent attention to your mental health, as is the case with your physical health, helps build emotional resilience over time.

Balancing Act

Remember that balancing your professional and personal life is an ongoing effort. It entails realizing the significance of self-renewal, regularly re-evaluating priorities, and establishing reasonable expectations. Being a mother makes it very important to balance your professional and home life. Parenting also becomes less challenging if you have support from your partner. Parenting that is collaborative, with open communication and shared responsibilities, is not limited to the first weeks and months. An ongoing plan will help to develop family relationships and adds to a happy family life.

Planning for Future Pregnancies

Many mothers have a question to ask: "In the coming years, should we have another baby, or should we not have another baby?" It's like having to choose between cake and more cake! Having the answer in hand lets you and your spouse make more informed decisions. Remember that planning a family is not simply about marking dates on a calendar; it is more like getting ready for the next installment of the ultimate adventure. Have you prepared yourself for the next round of restless nights? Another possibility is that you are contemplating a revolutionary method of birth control to prevent the stork from coming.

If you are thinking about growing your family, one of the most critical aspects to consider is the spacing of pregnancies. There is more to consider than how close your children will be in age to one another. Your family's life will be altered with the arrival of another child. Are you and your spouse prepared to take care of a baby again? What kind of reactions do you anticipate from your older child or children when they have to share your attention with a new baby?

Additionally, the impact of the timing of your pregnancies should not be overlooked. Some studies indicate that the spacing of your pregnancies may affect both the mother and the infant, even though you and your spouse may have preferences for the age gaps you would want your children to have (*Family Planning*, 2022).

Risks of Close Pregnancy Spacing

The time between the end of one pregnancy and the start of the next is called the pregnancy gap or the interpregnancy interval. Although there isn't a single agreed-upon meaning of what makes a "short" or "close" gap, most people agree it's less than 18 months. There are some risks for both the mother and the baby when the pregnancies are closer together than this. Researchers have found that starting a pregnancy within six months of having a live birth is linked to a higher risk of (*Family Planning*, 2022).

- preterm birth

- placental abruption (when the placenta peels off some or all of the inner wall of the uterus before birth)

- low weight at birth

- problems present at birth

- schizophrenia

- anemia in mothers

- uterine rupture

- breastfeeding challenges

Furthermore, second-born infants of mothers who had their pregnancies very close together may be at a higher risk of autism, according to new studies. The risk is most significant when the interval between pregnancies is shorter than 12 months (*Family Planning*, 2022).

Risks of Spacing Pregnancies Too Far Apart

Some research shows that extended gaps between pregnancies may raise the risk of pre-eclampsia in women without a history of it (*Family Planning*, 2022).

It's unclear why extended pregnancy gaps are unhealthy. Pregnancy may increase uterine capacity to support fetal development, although these physiological changes may fade with time.

Best Interval Between Pregnancies

Research proposes waiting at least 18–24 months but less than five years after a live birth before trying to conceive again to avoid pregnancy difficulties and other health issues. Considering the increased risk of infertility with age, people over 35 should wait 12 months before becoming pregnant again (*Family Planning*, 2022).

These risks and advice don't apply to couples who have experienced a miscarriage. After a miscarriage, you may try to conceive again immediately if you're healthy and ready.

When to have another child is a personal choice. Besides the health risks and rewards, you and your partner should consider other factors when planning your next pregnancy. There's no ideal moment to have another.

Use effective birth control until you decide to try to have another child. Even with careful preparation, conception is unpredictable. However, discussing dependable birth control methods until you are ready to conceive and knowing the hazards of timing your pregnancies will help you decide when to have children (Mayo Clinic Staff, 2022).

Birth Control Options

Parents often consider birth control after childbirth. If you wish to avoid pregnancy shortly after having your baby, use effective contraception. If you're not breastfeeding, use whichever contraception you choose. If you are breastfeeding, you need to be aware that contraception containing estrogen, such as the vaginal ring and the combination pill, may diminish breast milk production unless your infant is at least six weeks old and half bottle-fed. However, there are many more contraceptive options. Make sure you're not pregnant before starting to use contraception.

Most of the time, women are most likely to get pregnant two weeks before their period. Whether you are breastfeeding only, using formula, or doing a mix of the two, your periods will come back anywhere from six weeks to three months after giving birth. Some women may not get their periods again until they cut down on or stop breastfeeding. That being said, you might still get pregnant without knowing it. According to health experts, the best time to start using birth control after giving birth is about three weeks after the birth (Department of Health & Human Services, n.d.).

The different types of birth control are:

- the birth control implant, which works more than 99% of the time

- the birth control injection, which works more than 99% of the time

- the progesterone-only pill, which is 99% effective if taken correctly

- male condoms, which work 98% of the time if they are used properly

- female condoms, which work 95% of the time if they are used properly (NHS, 2018)

And finally, you can get an intrauterine device (IUD) or an intrauterine system (IUD) put in within 48 hours of giving birth. Both are more than 99% effective. If you don't get an IUD or IUS within 48 hours of giving birth, you'll probably be told to wait until four weeks after giving birth (NHS, 2018).

If you are breastfeeding, you can safely use mini pills, condoms, diaphragms, Depo-Provera or Depo-Ralovera injectables, the Implanon NXT implant, IUDs, and tubal ligation.

Note

Contraceptives containing estrogen are not advised for people who are breastfeeding because the estrogen is passed out of the body in breast milk, and no one knows how it will affect a baby. The emergency contraceptive pill is also not recommended. If a woman does use it, she shouldn't breastfeed for seven days afterward (Department of Health & Human Services, n.d.).

Return of Periods

Each woman has a different experience of when her periods start up again after giving birth. The timing of the first postpartum period can depend on things like breastfeeding and the method of birth control used. It's normal for periods to be unpredictable initially, so don't worry if they fluctuate occasionally.

Understanding the return of periods and investigating the many birth control choices available after giving birth are both essential components of family planning. Careful attention to factors such as pregnancy spacing, maternal health, family dynamics, and professional advice is vital when preparing for future pregnancies. This will help ensure your approach to growing your family is well-informed and healthy.

Learning, Resources, and Support

Beginning the parenting journey is a continuous learning process, and the ability to seek help is a characteristic of strength. As you navigate the ups and downs of parenthood, it is important to remember that the path of motherhood is enhanced by information, resources, and a supportive community.

When you become a mother, you and your child will learn and develop together. Explore a wide range of parenting books that provide insights into the development of children, the behavior of children, and successful parenting practices. There are a great deal of online platforms nowadays. Parenting courses are available on online platforms such as Coursera and Udemy. These courses cover various subjects, including developing mental skills and positive discipline.

You can also use many articles, ideas, and forums on websites such as Parenting.com, BabyCenter, and HealthyChildren.org. These websites allow parents to share their experiences and advise one another. What to Expect, The Wonder Weeks, and Peanut are examples of apps that link parents by providing them with advice, forums, and insights on their children's growth. By participating in local parenting groups, whether in person or online, you can connect with other parents who are going through the same things as you. Because of this, a shared feeling of community and experiences is created.

Several communities provide parenting programs that include a wide variety of subjects, ranging from prenatal care to the actions of toddlers. You can get information about the courses offered by contacting your area's community centers, hospitals, or parental groups.

Seeking out therapy or counseling is a helpful alternative to consider if the demands of parenting become overwhelming. Therapists who specialize in family relationships and parenting may provide individualized counseling services. Participating in a parenting support group, whether in-person or online, provides a forum where individuals may discuss their experiences, seek guidance, and get emotional support. Several organizations, such as Postpartum Support International and La Leche League, which provide support for nursing mothers, are excellent sources of information.

Importance of Continuous Growth

The road of parenting is dynamic, and the significance of unending education and development cannot be overstressed. Embrace the ever-changing nature of your position, maintain a sense of curiosity, and be willing to experiment with new approaches. Please remember that no universal method exists; every child is an individual.

The act of seeking and providing assistance is a process that reinforces the overall fabric of motherhood, which is a tapestry. The collective knowledge of the parenting community is an invaluable tool, and it can be obtained in various ways, including via books, internet resources, local organizations, and professional counsel. Always remember to appreciate the importance of learning, sharing, and developing as a parent as you continue on this road.

Conclusion

You are put under so much strain physically and mentally during pregnancy and labor, so it's no surprise your body and mind need time to heal and recover after such a life-changing event. Every mother will have a story to tell about her pregnancy, some of which will be positive, some negative, often emotional, and sometimes traumatic. This book has provided you with the most outstanding guidance so you can comprehend and manage your postpartum experience effectively.

So, let's be honest. When you were expecting your first child (or if you are currently pregnant), did anybody take the time to sit you down and give you an overall picture of what it would be like to go through the postpartum period? Most likely, the answer is no. If yes, you are one of the lucky few.

Moms-to-be have the right to know everything about labor and the time after giving birth. We often look for answers online, but it's only sometimes helpful. I have shared my story with you through these chapters to help you understand what happens and implement useful strategies in your life. My journey is different from my sister's. However, my feelings go up and down often, from being on cloud nine to crying sometimes. I'm always thinking about all the things I need to do. Since giving birth, my little bundle of joy has been very demanding, and I need to take care of both myself and my child. Every mom goes through this time, and it's okay!

I often see moms in a state similar to that of an airplane passenger, in that as a mother, you need to put on your own oxygen mask first before helping others. Take care of yourself; you're in charge of this journey.

Let's go over the most important things we have learned from our book and the key takeaways from each chapter.

Key Takeaways

As we reflect on our journey, we must highlight the significant points that represent the core of our postpartum health adventure. These include the following:

- **Understanding bodily changes postpartum:** After giving birth, our bodies undergo many changes that we must accept and enjoy. Know that the way to healing is different for every woman. If you are worried or unsure about changes in your body, you should talk to a professional.

- **Emotional and mental health:** Take care of your psychological and physical health simultaneously. Recognize that it is expected to have various emotions after giving birth. Foster an environment where people feel comfortable talking to one another and reaching out for help when needed.

- **Pain management:** Find out what works and what doesn't regarding postpartum pain management. Make an appointment with your doctor if you need help developing a plan to deal with your pain. Make sure to address both your pain and your general health.

- **Exercise:** Slowly include light activities as you settle into your postpartum routine. Put your energy into things that will make you more robust, flexible, and fit. Talk to your doctor before beginning an exercise program if you have health concerns.

- **Understanding nutrition and recovery:** Eat healthily after giving birth to aid with the healing process. Consider what you need to eat, particularly the minerals and vitamins necessary for recovery. Staying adequately hydrated is essential for maintaining good health and wellness.

- **Importance of proper breastfeeding:** Acknowledge the value of using correct breastfeeding methods. Consult with healthcare professionals or lactation specialists for advice. Ensure your mental and physical well-being when you breastfeed.

- **Newborn care:** Learn the fundamentals of caring for your baby, including feeding, sleeping, and personal cleanliness. Accept that a learning curve will be involved in meeting a newborn's specific demands. Create a community of people who can relate so you can talk to them and get their advice.

- **Self-care:** After giving birth, it's important to make self-care a regular part of your schedule. Take time for yourself and remember how important it is to relax and unwind. Share your self-care requirements with those close to you who can help.

- **Parenting with confidence:** Familiarity with your newborn's wants and indications may help build your confidence. Have faith in your gut as a parent and ask for help when needed. Have a good attitude and be resilient as you embark on the adventure of motherhood.

These essential lessons will help you navigate the complex postpartum period and promote holistic healing, well-being, and confident parenting.

By emphasizing physical recovery, emotional well-being, and confident parenting, this book has described the postpartum experience with the aim of guiding new parents. It has taken a comprehensive approach to postpartum healing, including physical changes, emotional issues, and self-care, and has provided practical advice on pain management, exercise, nutrition, breastfeeding, baby care, and parenting confidence to promote resilience and positivity. This thorough guide has been designed to help people negotiate the changing postpartum journey with knowledge, compassion, and confidence.

The information presented on these pages has shown us how important it is to have an excellent knowledge of the postpartum period. Remember to rejoice in the miracle of childbirth and what your body has accomplished. It is not easy to carry a baby for nine months and then go through the birthing process! You have earned every single inch and mark, so celebrate that instead of fretting about what the mirror or scales say.

A Call to Action

Do something for yourself. Celebrate successes and recognize obstacles as you reflect on your journey. Also, the most crucial thing is to seek the assistance you need. You're not alone. Start your postpartum journey with confidence. It is essential to acknowledge the significance of self-care, the comprehension of changes in the body, and the cultivation of emotional well-being. Manage discomfort, exercise gently, eat well, and value breastfeeding and baby care. This prompt urges you to build a support network, express your needs, and embrace motherhood. Your path is unique—be resilient, learn, and be optimistic. You should use the postpartum phase for good and welcome its changes.

Share the information: Tell your loved ones about your postpartum transformation. Let's highlight the entire experience of postpartum recovery to develop a helpful community. Encourage others to read the book's advice on healthy living, emotional resilience, and confident parenting. Your voice matters. **Consider reviewing this book on Amazon or your favorite bookshop. Doing so will help the growing network of postpartum women seeking knowledge and support to navigate this transformative path with information and confidence.**

Lastly, most new parents fear making mistakes. But remember that there is no "right way" or "one way" to be a parent or care for your infant. Trusting yourself and your instincts is crucial. Nobody knows your child better than you!

Appendix:

Baby Food—Six to Twelve Months

During your baby's first year, their nutritional needs will change. When they are about six months old, most babies are ready to start solid foods along with breast milk or infant formula. Your baby will drink less breast milk or infant formula as they eat more solid foods, although the milk is still essential. Once your baby reaches the age of six months, they will typically nurse around five to six times each day. It would be best if you continue to breastfeed your child while you are transitioning to solid meals. When you breastfeed for extended periods, you and your baby will reap additional benefits. Breastfeeding babies don't require other milk.

After six months, it is advised that newborns be given water to taste, and they should be given a few sips of it. Babies don't need juice; however, you can give them 100% juice in an open cup as a meal or snack. If they Consuming more than 1/2 cup (125 milliliters) of juice daily can reduce your baby's appetite, increase their risk of dental decay, and provide them with a significant amount of sugar they do not need. Your child should not consume juice that has not been pasteurized.

Signs Your Baby Is Ready for Solids

Swallowing food is different from consuming milk. A baby's mouth is built to suckle and swallow before they are six months old. Your baby will learn to move food from the front of their mouth to the back so they can safely eat at around six months old. At this point, solid foods can be slowly added. When your baby reaches the following milestones, it's time to introduce solid foods:

- They need little assistance to sit up.

- When they aren't hungry, they can move their heads away, demonstrating excellent control of their neck and head.

- When given food, they can open their mouth.

Around six months of age, when your baby displays all the signs of readiness, you may start introducing solid foods (*Starting Solid Foods*, n.d.).

Critical Guidelines for Introducing Solid Foods

Your baby might need a few tries before getting used to eating solid things. Remember that they are trying new ways to use their mouth, tongue, and throat. It can be fun and messy for you and your baby when they start eating solid foods. To learn, babies like to touch their food and try to eat on their own.

- **Developmental readiness:** Ensure your infant is ready for solids before starting them. These may include sitting up with some help, displaying an interest in eating, and reducing the tongue-thrust reflex.

- **Start with single foods:** Rice and oatmeal are iron-fortified single-ingredient infant cereals. Starting with these helps you detect allergies and sensitivities.

- **One food at a time:** Introduce a new foods (fruits / vegetable) every three to five days. This spacing lets you watch for allergies in your infant. A response makes it easy to identify the cause.

- **Watch for allergies:** Rashes, hives, vomiting, diarrhea, and fussiness may indicate allergies. Consult your doctor immediately if these symptoms arise.

- **Avoid common allergens first:** Peanuts, tree nuts, dairy, eggs, and shellfish should not be introduced unless your doctor approves. To test your baby's responses, introduce these foods one at a time in small quantities.

- **Texture and consistency matter:** Start with smooth and pureed textures, then lumpy and mashed as your baby becomes used to eating. This phase will improve oral and motor skills.

- **Maintain feeding comfort:** Be happy and calm throughout meals. Comfortable and supported babies are more likely to try new foods.

- **Watch for your baby's cues:** Pay attention to your baby's feeding signals. Respect their indifference or walk away signals. Please do not force them to eat.

- **Introducing table foods gradually:** Start transitioning your infant from purees to soft, age-appropriate table meals around their first birthday. Encourage self-feeding for independence and fine motor skills.

- **Regular doctor visits:** Inform your doctor about your baby's feedings. Regular checkups allow you to address problems, obtain dietary advice, and safeguard your baby's health.

Suitable Foods

Foods at Six Months

- Single-grain baby cereals (rice, oatmeal)

- Pureed fruits (apples, pears, whatever you like)

- Pureed vegetables (sweet potatoes, carrots)

- Single-ingredient purees

Foods at Seven to Eight Months

- Mashed or finely chopped soft foods

- Bananas, avocados

- Well-cooked and finely diced vegetables

- Small portions of delicate meats

Foods at Nine to Ten Months

- Increase the texture with soft finger foods

- Introduce yogurt and cheese

- Incorporate finely shredded or minced protein sources

Foods at Eleven to Twelve Months

- Gradual transition to more textured foods

- Introducing small portions of family meals (finely chopped)

- Explore a variety of grains, proteins, and fruits

The transition to solids is gradual and personalized. Follow your baby's cues, praise their curiosity, and enjoy this fascinating food adventure!

Sample Meal Plan From Six to Twelve Months

Six Months

- **Breakfast:** Single-grain cereal with breast milk or formula

- **Lunch:** Pureed apples or pears

- **Dinner:** Pureed sweet potatoes or carrots

Seven to Eight Months

- **Breakfast:** Mashed bananas mixed with baby cereal

- **Lunch:** Finely chopped avocados

- **Dinner:** Soft vegetable puree with small portions of finely diced chicken

Nine to Ten Months

- **Breakfast:** Finger-sized pieces of well-cooked scrambled eggs

- **Lunch:** Yogurt with mashed berries

- **Dinner:** Quinoa mixed with finely shredded cheese and steamed vegetables

Eleven to Twelve Months

- **Breakfast:** Oatmeal with diced fruits

- **Lunch:** Mini sandwiches with mashed beans

- **Dinner:** Family meal of finely chopped pasta with tomato sauce, minced meat, and mixed vegetables

Nutritional Considerations

Your baby's growth and well-being depend on appropriate nutrition from six to twelve months. Some important nutritional considerations are as follows:

- Iron is essential for brain and body growth. Fortified single-grain baby cereals, well-cooked proteins, and pureed beans are iron-rich diets for babies. Diversity in iron sources prevents iron-deficiency anemia.

- Brain growth and nervous system support depend on healthy fats. Add avocados, mashed bananas, and yogurt to your baby's diet. The absorption of fat-soluble vitamins A, D, E, and K requires these lipids.

- As well as providing nutrition, providing different foods exposes your child to varied tastes and sensations. Include diverse fruits, veggies, grains, and proteins. Variety helps build taste preferences and supplies critical minerals.

- Calcium and vitamin D are vital for bone health. Introduce dairy food like yogurt and cheese, and expose your child to sunshine for natural vitamin D synthesis. If your baby is not consuming dairy, consult healthcare professionals to explore alternative sources.

- When your baby is eating a more varied diet, offer fiber-rich meals such as finely chopped fruits, veggies, and whole grains. Fiber aids digestion and nutrition balance.

- Water should be introduced slowly when your infant starts eating solids, even if breast milk or formula is the primary source of hydration. Hydration is crucial for health.

Remember, each baby has different dietary demands. I hope that the journey of your baby's culinary experience is as enjoyable for you as it is for them, and that each meal is a time of connection and sustenance for you and your baby.

References

Andrus, P. (2022, November 3). *The best schedule for your baby*. Parents. https://www.parents.com/baby/sleep/schedule/the-best-schedule-for-your-baby/

Aoki, C., Imai, K., Owaki, T., Kobayashi-Nakano, T., Ushida, T., Iitani, Y., Nakamura, N., Kajiyama, H., & Kotani, T. (2022). The possible effects of zinc supplementation on postpartum depression and anemia. *Medicina*, *58*(6), 731. https://doi.org/10.3390/medicina58060731

Attachment: A connection for life. (n.d.). Caring for Kids. https://caringforkids.cps.ca/handouts/pregnancy-and-babies/attachment

Baby blues after pregnancy. (n.d.). March of Dimes. https://www.marchofdimes.org/find-support/topics/postpartum/baby-blues-after-pregnancy

BetterHelp Editorial Team. (2023, September 28). *Why self care matters for moms*. BetterHelp https://www.betterhelp.com/advice/mindfulness/why-self-care-is-important-for-mothers/

Bonding with your baby. (n.d.). Nemours KidsHealth. https://kidshealth.org/en/parents/bonding.html

Brianna. (2020, January 30). *How to avoid the comparison trap*. Mastering Mom Life. https://masteringmomlife.com/dangers-of-comparing-your-child-to-others/

Brown-Worsham, S. (2023, January 21). *20 things to know about your postpartum body*. Parents. https://www.parents.com/pregnancy/my-body/postpartum/your-postpartum-body-what-to-expect-and-what-to-do/

Catholic Health Initiatives. (n.d.). *The fourth trimester*. CHI Health. https://www.chihealth.com/en/services/maternity/postpartu m-care/the-fourth-trimester.html

Centers for Disease Control and Prevention. (n.d.-a). *About mental health*. https://www.cdc.gov/mentalhealth/learn/index.htm

Centers for Disease Control and Prevention. (n.d.-b). *Depression among women*. https://www.cdc.gov/reproductivehealth/depression/index.ht m

Centers for Disease Control and Prevention. (n.d.-c). *Maternal diet*. https://www.cdc.gov/breastfeeding/breastfeeding-special-circumstances/diet-and-micronutrients/maternal-diet.html

Cradlewise Staff. (2023, August 23). *Matrescence: The complex reality of your birth as a mother*. Cradlewise. https://cradlewise.com/blog/matrescence-your-birth-as-a-mother

Cristol, H. (n.d.). *Alternatives to breastfeeding*. WebMD. https://www.webmd.com/parenting/baby/features/breastfeed ing-alternatives

De Bellefonds, C. (2023, July 25). *Diastasis recti (Ab separation)*. What to Expect. https://www.whattoexpect.com/pregnancy/pregnancy-health/diastasis-recti-and-pregnancy/

Department of Health & Human Services. (n.d.). *Contraception after giving birth*. Better Health Channel. https://www.betterhealth.vic.gov.au/health/healthyliving/cont raception-after-giving-birth

Enger, L., & Hurst, N. M. (2023, May 5). *Patient education: Pumping breast milk (beyond the basics)*. UpToDate.

https://www.uptodate.com/contents/pumping-breast-milk-beyond-the-basics

Exercise during pregnancy. (n.d.). March of Dimes. https://www.marchofdimes.org/find-support/topics/pregnancy/exercise-during-pregnancy

Family planning: Get the facts about pregnancy spacing. (2022, December 2). Mayo Clinic. https://www.mayoclinic.org/healthy-lifestyle/getting-pregnant/in-depth/family-planning/art-20044072

The 4th trimester: embracing the bond between mother and baby. (2023, June 20). Clear Chiropractic. https://www.getclearchiropractic.com/the-4th-trimester-embracing-the-bond-between-mother-and-baby/

Grao. (2019, May 2). *15 ingredients speed up wound healing.* NS Healthcare. https://www.ns-healthcare.com/news/15-ingredients-speed-up-wound-healing-7179127/

A guide for first-time parents. (n.d.). Nemours KidsHealth. https://kidshealth.org/en/parents/guide-parents.html

Hanh, T. N. (n.d.). *Thich Nhat Hanh quotes.* https://www.goodreads.com/quotes/119873-life-can-be-found-only-in-the-present-moment-th

Healthdirect Australia. (n.d.-b). *Complementary therapy during pregnancy.* Pregnancy, Birth & Baby. https://www.pregnancybirthbaby.org.au/complementary-therapy-during-pregnancy

Healthdirect Australia. (n.d.-a). *Burping, wind and colic in babies.* Pregnancy, Birth & Baby. https://www.pregnancybirthbaby.org.au/burping-wind-and-colic-in-babies

Horsager-Boehrer, R. (2022, October 11). *6 ways to embrace a more positive body image during and after pregnancy.* UT Southwestern Medical Center. https://utswmed.org/medblog/perinatal-body-dissatisfaction/

Iavarone , K. (2023, March 29). *Understanding postpartum insomnia.* Medical News Today. https://www.medicalnewstoday.com/articles/postpartum-insomnia

Johns Hopkins Medicine. (n.d.). *Baby blues and postpartum depression: Mood disorders and pregnancy.* https://www.hopkinsmedicine.org/health/wellness-and-prevention/postpartum-mood-disorders-what-new-moms-need-to-know

Karges, C. (2023, February 21). *Postpartum period and body image.* Eating Disorder Hope. https://www.eatingdisorderhope.com/information/pregorexia/postpartum-period-and-body-image

Karp, H. (n.d.). *Newborn sleep tips and habits.* Happiest Baby. https://www.happiestbaby.com/blogs/baby/baby-sleep-habits

Kinghorn, K. (2023, February 6). *Managing postpartum depression: Coping strategies for new mothers.* Therapy Utah. https://therapyutah.org/managing-post-partum-depression/

Latch and position. (n.d.). The MotHERS Program. https://www.themothersprogram.ca/infant-care/breastfeeding/latch-and-position

Lindberg , S. (2020, July 31). *Postpartum diet plan: Tips for healthy eating after giving birth.* Healthline. https://www.healthline.com/health/postpartum-diet

Maas, E. (2023, May 25). *Getting mentally fit after baby: 7 ways for busy new mothers to prioritize their mental health.* Scrubbing In by BaylorScott&White Health. https://www.bswhealth.com/blog/getting-mentally-fit-after-baby

Managing stress in early parenthood. (n.d.). Centre of Perinatal Excellence (COPE). https://www.cope.org.au/new-parents/emotional-health-new-parents/managing-stress/

Mayo Clinic Staff. (2022, December 2). *Family planning: Get the facts about pregnancy spacing.* Mayo Clinic. https://www.mayoclinic.org/healthy-lifestyle/getting-pregnant/in-depth/family-planning/art-20044072

McCallum, K. (2021, February 17). *Postpartum exercise: What to know about exercising after pregnancy.* Houston Methodist. https://www.houstonmethodist.org/blog/articles/2021/feb/postpartum-exercise-what-to-know-about-exercising-after-pregnancy/

McDermott, A. (2023, May 24). *12 essential oils to help heal or prevent stretch marks.* Healthline. https://www.healthline.com/health/essential-oils-for-stretch-marks

Nall, R. (2023, June 23). *Does bromelain have any health benefits?* Medical News Today. https://www.medicalnewstoday.com/articles/323783

National Childbirth Trust. (2023, November 22). *What is the fourth trimester?* https://www.nct.org.uk/baby-toddler/emotional-and-social-development/what-fourth-trimester

NHS. (2018, October 3). *When can I use contraception after having a baby?* https://www.nhs.uk/conditions/contraception/when-contraception-after-baby/

O'Connor, A. (2022, September 5). *How to get a proper breastfeeding latch* What to Expect. https://www.whattoexpect.com/poor-breastfeeding-latch.aspx

Olsson, R. (2022, March 21). *7 breastfeeding problems and how to fix them.* Banner Health. https://www.bannerhealth.com/healthcareblog/advise-me/7-common-breastfeeding-challenges-and-how-to-solve-them

Park Academy Childcare. (2022, May 1). *Tips for choosing a childcare provider.* https://www.parkchildcare.ie/tips-for-choosing-a-childcare-provider/

Positioning. (n.d.). La Leche League International. https://llli.org/breastfeeding-info/positioning/

Postpartum care for mom: Tips for healing and comfort. (n.d.). Geisinger. https://www.geisinger.org/patient-care/conditions-treatments-specialty/self-care-during-the-postpartum-period

Postpartum nutrition: What to eat after you give birth? (2022, January 25). High Country Doulas. https://www.highcountrydoulas.com/blog/2022/1/18/postpartum-nutrition

Postpartum pain management. (n.d.). Newton-Wellesley Hospital, Mass General Brigham. https://www.nwh.org/maternity-guide/postpartum-guide/postpartum-chapter-2/postpartum-care-pain-management

Potential postpartum complications. (n.d.). Beaumont Health. https://www.beaumont.org/services/womens-services/maternity/after-pregnancy/moms-health/potential-complications

Pregnancy and body changes: Embracing your evolving self-image. (n.d.). Ovum Woiman & Child Speciality Hospital. https://ovumhospitals.com/blog/pregnancy-and-body-changes-embracing-your-evolving-self-image

Pump and dump: Is it necessary after drinking? (n.d.). Medela. https://www.medela.us/breastfeeding/articles/pump-and-dump-is-it-necessary-after-drinking

Recognizing newborn illnesses. (2023, October). Familydoctor.org. https://familydoctor.org/recognizing-newborn-illnesses/

Recovering from delivery (postpartum recovery). (2023, November). Familydoctor.org. https://familydoctor.org/recovering-from-delivery/

Reinagel, M. (2019, December 5). *Top 5 nutrients for postpartum recovery.* Scientific American.

https://www.scientificamerican.com/article/top-5-nutrients-for-postpartum-recovery/

Shen, Y., Huang, L., Zou, Y., Su, D., He, M., Fang, Y., Zhao, D., Wang, W., & Zhang, R. (2022). Intake of vitamin b12 and folate and biomarkers of nutrient status of women within two years postpartum. *Nutrients*, *14*(18), 3869. https://doi.org/10.3390/nu14183869

Shiraz, Z. (2022, July 6). Workout tips: 19 best exercises for repairing diastasis recti postpartum. *Hindustan Times*. https://www.hindustantimes.com/lifestyle/health/workout-tips-19-best-exercises-for-repairing-diastasis-recti-postpartum-101657105935868.html

Soni, S. (2023, September 7). *5 hygiene tips for healthy newborn baby care*. Littloo. https://littloo.in/blogs/best-baby-blog/5-essential-hygiene-tips-for-healthy-newborn-baby-care

Squillace, M. (2023, November 20). Your guide to pumping *at work*. What to Expect. https://www.whattoexpect.com/first-year/breastfeeding/tips-pumping-work/

Starting solid foods: 6–12 months. (n.d.). Healthy Parents Healthy Children. https://www.healthyparentshealthychildren.ca/im-a-parent/older-babies-6-12-months/feeding-starting-solid-foods/

Stewart, K. (2018, April 18). *Natural remedies for postpartum*. Doula Wisdom. https://www.doulawisdom.com/blog/natural-remedies-for-postpartum

Thompson, M. (2023, November 28). *What is postpartum depression?* Metropolitan Pediatrics. https://www.metropediatrics.com/pediatric-blog/what-is-postpartum-depression/

3 amazing ways to be present with your baby. (2021, October 20). Baby Tour Guide. https://www.babytourguide.com/2021/10/21/3-amazing-ways-to-be-present-with-your-baby/

3 ways to build a support network as a mother. (n.d.). Ovl Collection. https://ovlcollection.com/blogs/news/build-your-village-the-three-components-of-a-healthy-village-in-motherhood

Udechuku, A. (2021, August 2). *Postnatal depression, postnatal anxiety or normal adjustment after birth?* Glow Clinic. https://glowclinic.com.au/postnatal-depression-pna-or-normal-adjustment-to-parenting/

U.S. Department of Health and Human Services and U.S. Department of Agriculture. (2015, December). *2015–2020 dietary guidelines.* https://health.gov/our-work/nutrition-physical-activity/dietary-guidelines/previous-dietary-guidelines/2015

Warning signs of postpartum health problems. (n.d.). March of Dimes. https://www.marchofdimes.org/find-support/topics/postpartum/warning-signs-postpartum-health-problems

What to expect in the fourth trimester. (n.d.). Australian Birth Stories. https://australianbirthstories.com/postpartum/what-to-expect-in-the-fourth-trimester/

Wolf, K. (2019, November 22). *The postpartum diet.* Mama Strut by PELV-ICE. https://mamastrut.com/the-postpartum-diet

Working moms: Childcare options and getting ready. (n.d.). Medela. https://www.medela.us/breastfeeding/articles/working-moms-childcare-options-and-getting-ready

WOW Parenting. (2019, May 15). *10 life-changing time management tips for working moms.* https://wowparenting.com/blog/time-management-tips-for-working-women/